Plant based diet
Meal Plan

document, including but not limited to errors, omissions or inaccuracies.

Table of Content

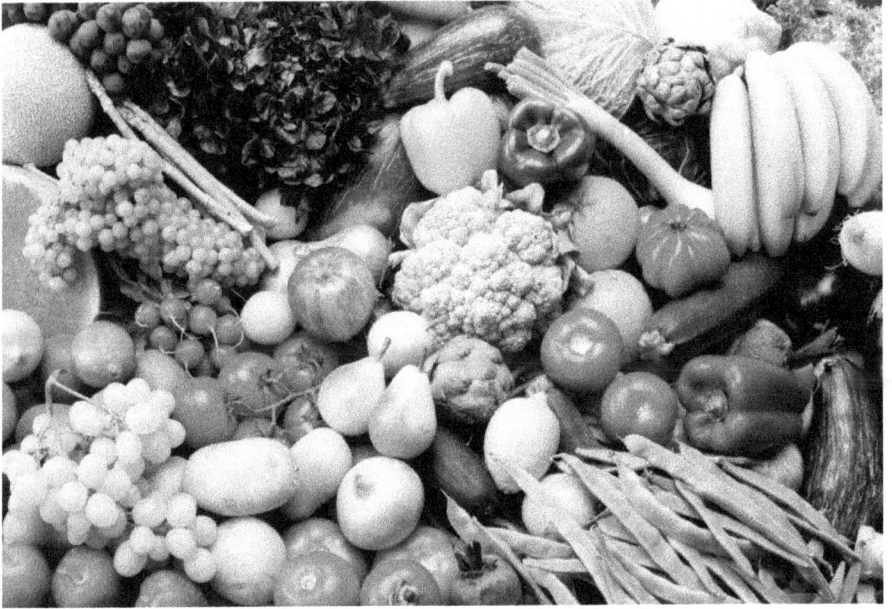

Introduction

Like most people who change plants, I wondered if the food would be enough. I also worried about finding uninspiring and restrictive plant foods, mainly because of the belief that plant products meant eating boring and tasteless salads. So, I worked a little bit to learn how to make healthy planet products amazing. I followed the chef's training for an intuitive vegetable-based cuisine, which involves learning to cook according to your intuitions as a chef, without using recipes. Since I wanted to make sure .I have everything my body needs to grow, I went back to school to learn essential nutrition, focusing on a natural approach to healthy living.

I had never had so much fun cooking and eating before. I never feel limited or private; in reverse .I feel free, discovering unlimited possibilities with new flavors and new combinations of flavors and constantly adding new and exciting foods and meals to my recipe list. After moving on to a plant-based lifestyle, I have more energy; I lost weight without trying; and I have no chronic gas or digestion problems .I have had in the past. I didn't realize how bad I felt until I felt better.

This is how my path to plants developed, but I know that each path is different because our food experiences are different. The way we eat is very personal. Food not only feeds our body, it has the power to make life more enjoyable. Food is closely linked to cultures and social life and our taste buds force us to seek happiness and satisfaction from the food we eat. Maintaining a plant lifestyle can be difficult in a meat-centered, comfortoriented society. Most people are intimidated by the idea of stopping eating well and learning to prepare new and strange dishes from those who know little or nothing and sometimes cannot even pronounce. And if you eat plants it's not natural, it's hard to get excited about the countless vegan cookbooks and blogs and trust existing plants.

This is where the book is different. The food plan and recipes in this book are designed to teach you how to prepare the best vegetable meals so that the meal itself becomes an incentive. Since no matter what the reason for switching to plants is, it is enough to include more vegetables in the diet, lose ten pounds stubborn, look slim for this special occasion, make long-term health changes as prescribed by a doctor find relief from chronic diseases and symptoms or, like me, they reduce the carbon footprint by reducing meat and dairy products; In fact, if the taste of the food you eat does not excite you, you cannot maintain this way of eating for up to three weeks.

I decided to arm myself with culinary education, but it's not that far from success with this diet. Using the knowledge and techniques that have helped me and my numerous clients, I have carefully developed these recipes to study different dishes thanks to quick and easy meals that are practical after work or on a busy night. I was also inspired by kitchens around the world, so I can discover your new favorite food, food or recipe by expanding your vocabulary and food experience. Additionally, the threeweek meal plan includes daily menus and shopping lists to show you exactly how to make this diet work for you and help you stay on track. You will find a clear guide and a solid plan of action to switch to a completely nutritious vegetable diet, with a constant focus on delicious and healthy foods. You can also prepare meals that meat lovers will fall in love with.

Finally, the wonderful thing about eating and enjoying plants is that in three weeks you will start to see and feel their healing power. Your complexion will appear more radiant, digestion will improve, you will have more energy, you will think better and you will sleep better .If you follow this long-term diet, you should find that your immune system is more resistant, your mood is more balanced, your life is thinner and your mind calms down when you make decisions.

What is this plant-based diet?

All plant foods and diets are sometimes called the WFPB diet; Although many dietitians and doctors have some differences in the list of plant diets, they all agree on one thing: a plant diet or WFPB is more than a diet First of all, it is a lifestyle.

It is a lifestyle that means different things to different people, because people also determine which vegetable diet is for them while some people leave room for animal products like eggs and milk; others decide not to allow any type of animal products in their diet.

However, most people's plant based diet has some characteristics that make them generally accepted by nutritionists, doctors and individuals. These characteristics are

- The foods you focus on are basically plants like vegetables, fruits, legumes, seeds, whole grains and nuts
- Is there a limitation or a total ban on products of animal origin (depending on the person)
- This diet helps to focus on the quality of the food consumed and many followers of the plant diet are 100% organic food and are obtained locally
- All dietary plant products are whole without processing (or very little processing, if any)

These basic reasons mean that this diet is sometimes confused with a vegan or vegetarian diet; although they have their similarities, they still have their peculiarities.

What is the difference?

Vegan diet: people who follow a vegan diet stay away from any form of animal products such as shellfish, honey, meat, eggs, milk and poultry.

Vegetarians: there are two types of vegetarians; there are those who eat dairy products, seafood. There are also vegetarians who eliminate poultry and meat from their diet.

Plant-based diet: the plant-based diet is quite flexible Many advocates consume plant-based foods, but animal products are not potentially lethal taboos (although some think so) Some people follow a comprehensive plan-based diet, while others eat milk, eggs, poultry, meat and seafood.

Plant or plant based diets (as some people call it) are diets that focus on healthy plant based foods.

Are plant-based diets the best solution?

Some people have had a reason to ask me if vegetable diets are really a good option because there are also health benefits that can be obtained from sources that are not exclusive.

It's true, but you have nothing to lose if you follow an exclusively vegetable diet.

Thanks to the vegetable diet, you get the necessary nutrients, such as vitamins, fats, proteins, minerals and carbohydrates for a healthy diet and body, as well as being rich in nutrients and fiber.For those who omit all forms of animal products in their diet, they must take certain nutrients, such as B12, so that their body can get all the nutrients they need.

Some told me that I would stick to this diet, but my options are limited.

There is no greater lie than that Did you know that you can prepare cocktails, purees, pizzas and other delicious and delicious dishes that will make your palate more desirable? Plus, they're all healthy and nutritious plant products! You can't have it better.

Even if you continue with this diet, you can be sure that you have all the necessary nutrients in your food, even if it is a plant-based diet .Herbal products ensure that your body does not lack the minerals necessary for the healthy development and growth of the body.

What about vitamin B12?

Vitamin B12 is an essential nutrient that the body needs to keep blood cells and nerves active and healthy .Thanks to this vitamin, the body can protect itself from a serious state of anemia, known as megaloblastic anemia, and rejuvenates the body so that it does not wear out and does not tire easily People with low levels of vitamin B12 can pass out due to fatigue.

This particular vitamin is one of the few vitamins obtained from animal products; You can find dairy products like milk or margarine.If you use a plant-based diet that does not contain animal products, you can easily get tired or pass out.

A good way to get this vitamin is to take vitamin B $_{12}$ in the form of food supplements

Don't worry, even people who don't follow a plant-based diet, such as the elderly, pregnant women and others with vitamin B $_{12}$ deficiency , take these supplements With age, the body has difficulty absorbing this vitamin, so the doctor may prescribe this drug.

What happens to Omega-3 fatty acid?

Omega-3 fatty acids are very important for the body .It is known to help the body fight inflammation, increase the body's resistance and prevent autoimmune diseases, prevent cancer, help the body's mental health, relieve anxiety and depression and help the brain develop a fetus , prevents Alzheimer's disease, reduces the risk of ADHD and asthma in children and reduces the risk of heart disease.

Omega-3 fatty acids are usually found in blue fish (in large quantities), but this does not mean that they cannot be found in other seeds and nuts. If you follow a plant-based diet, you can get it from other sources, such as hemp seeds, nuts, soybeans, chia seeds, ground flax seeds, flax seeds and their oils Omega-3 fatty acids are also found in algae oil and perilla oil.

PLANT-BASED DIET PRINTER

Before moving on to balanced food programs and delicious recipes, let's take some time to learn and understand the principles and science of a plant-based diet. You may be interested in getting started, but in the long run it's worth finding out why and what we do. It will also save you time, because you will begin to understand how to prepare a balanced and delicious meal, instead of always following plans and recipes. In the first chapter we will see the relationship between a plant-based diet and your health; then we will move on to the balanced plant nutrition division; and then I will give you many tips and tricks on how to set up a plant-based kitchen.

PLANTS AND YOURS HEALTH

Unfortunately, chronic diseases like cancer and heart disease are very common in the United States. There is good evidence that changing eating habits can help prevent chronic diseases and a diet rich in meat and dairy products is associated with some important health complications, such as heart disease and diabetes. Numerous meat and dairy compounds (such as casein, nitrite, saturated fat, cholesterol, heme iron and arachidonic acid) are involved as possible culprits for this combination.

All this has aroused a growing interest in the diet of plants for health reasons, because plant foods are a rich source of nutrients and compounds that help us protect ourselves from chronic diseases. Before discussing what to eat to support this new lifestyle, it is necessary to further examine the role that plants play in controlling weight loss and promoting a healthier life.

Plants as medicine

One of the most important choices you can make for your health is to eat more fresh fruit and vegetables, whole grains, beans, nuts, seeds, herbs and spices. Incorporating more of these products into your life has powerful effects.

Plant-based diets are rich in dietary fiber, magnesium, folic acid, vitamins C and E, iron and phyto chemicals. They also have a lower calorific value and they are less saturated fat and cholesterol than other diets. Vegetarians generally have a lower risk of cardiovascular disease, obesity, type 2 diabetes and some types of cancer.

Cardiovascular diseases

Heart disease is the most important cause of American death .Dietary recommendations for people at risk of cardiovascular disease include a reduction in saturated fat, cholesterol, refined carbohydrates and sugar and an increase in fiber, antioxidants, omega-3 and monounsaturated fats. The best way to achieve this is through a vegetable diet (eating vegetables, whole grains, nuts, seeds, legumes and fruits).

In studies, vegans have lower cardiovascular disease rates than carnivores and even vegetarians: low blood pressure, low LDL cholesterol (bad type), low triglyceride levels, low total serum cholesterol and apolipoprotein B levels (transported cholesterol) by lipoproteins in the blood and apolipoproteins are a component of many lipoproteins involved in atherosclerosis and cardiovascular disease, reduce systolic and diastolic blood pressure and also reduce the incidence of hypertension.

Vegetarians generally have a lower incidence of hypertension, probably due to the high potassium intake of vegetables, fruit, whole grains and legumes. Blood pressure is related to the percentage of sodium to potassium in your body. Although a common recommendation for people with hypertension is to reduce salt intake, it has not been shown that it has a significant impact on blood pressure control. Another key to this equation is to increase the potassium side of the compound. The average consumption for a typical American is 2: 1, which means that you are twice as much of sodium than the desired potassium. The ideal ratio is 1: 5, so reducing the salt (sodium chloride) doesn't take it far enough. It is necessary to eat more plant foods to increase the potassium side of the balance.

The diet of plants significantly increases the intake of protective nutrients (such as antioxidants) and phytochemicals (compounds in plants that are useful to us), minimizing the intake of risky compounds that are involved in various chronic diseases. This does not mean that vegans are immune from disease: inheritance and other environmental and lifestyle factors are also involved. But a plant-based diet offers the best chance of avoiding risks and helps develop a strong immune system to face any challenge beyond your control.

Cancer

Cancer is the second leading cause of death in the United States. Whole plant foods, i.e. those as close as possible to their natural state, are rich in powerful antioxidants to fight cancer and nutrients that stimulate the immune system and naturally have a low content of saturated fat and a high fiber content many more legumes (seeds, peas and beans), more fruit and vegetables in total, more fiber and more vitamin C than omnivores. These foods and their nutrients are those that have proven to be particularly protective against cancer. The plant-based diet also reduces foods associated with an increased risk of cancer, including dairy products, eggs, red meat and processed meat.

Race

The risk factors for stroke are similar to cardiovascular disease: high cholesterol, hypertension and obesity. Since a plant-based diet improves all three, it is a good way to offset the risk.

Alzheimer's disease and dementia

While the onset of Alzheimer's disease and dementia are mainly caused by heredity, a nutrient-rich plant diet offers our bodies the best chance of staying healthy for as long as possible. One of the factors that can accelerate the onset of dementia is oxidative stress, an imbalance between the level of free radicals in the body and the ability to neutralize its harmful effects through antioxidants (Free radicals damage cell membranes and other structures, including DNA) .Plants are the richest source of antioxidants in the diet and can help reduce this damage.

Recommendations to delay the onset and delay the progression of Alzheimer's disease often include the consumption of fish and shellfish, in the case of omega-3 fatty acids. However, research also indicates that toxins, heavy metals and c is nerve cells ANC is at n contributing and contributing to neurodegeneraci on. Since fish and crustaceans are inevitably rich in mercury and other toxins that pollute our oceans, such as plastic, it makes more sense to look for virgin sources of omega-3, such as flaxseed and chia.

One of the first questions I ask myself when people talk about their parents starting to show signs of dementia is whether they are getting enough vitamin B_{12} and folic acid. A deficiency in one of these nutrients causes symptoms that mimic dementia. Folic acid can be easily obtained from plant foods, but the density of nutrients needed to maintain a healthy body and mind is not always a priority in our diet. When the metabolism of the elderly slows down, they need more of these nutrients, not less. As we age, our bodies are less able to get vitamin B_{12} from our food, so that the government's recommendations are people over 50 take a supplement of B_{12}, regardless of whether they eat foods of animal origin.

Diabetes

The main dietary recommendations for diabetes include reducing the glycemic load (general nutritional potential for increasing blood sugar levels) and taking saturated fat, increasing fiber intake and the use of cinnamon. It has been studied to obtain possible benefits in controlling blood sugar levels. This can be easily achieved through a plant-based diet. Many people with pre-diabetes and people with type 2 diabetes find that their blood sugar levels are much easier to control when consuming a plant-based diet.

PLANTS AND COMMON INFLAMMATION

Studies of the relationship between arthritis and diet have shown that people on a plant diet show a significant reduction in morning stiffness, joint pain, swelling and inflammatory compounds in the blood. This is probably due to the fact that the plant-based diet increases the intake of anti-inflammatory foods and reduces the intake of inflammatory compounds from foods of animal origin. There may also be a connection with a bacterium called Yersinia, which is found in contaminated pigs, which can cause chronic inflammation. Worse still, vegans generally have a lower body weight than those who eat meat, which puts less pressure on the joints.

FOODS THAT INCREASE INFLAMMATION

Meat, fish and eggs are rich sources of arachidonic acid, which is a precursor to inflammatory compounds (prostaglandins and leukotrienes). A low arachidonic acid diet has been shown to help relieve arthritis symptoms. Advanced glycation end products (AGE) are inflammatory toxins that appear when food is heated, cooked, fried or pasteurized. They are formed mainly in foods of animal origin, because the reaction is caused by protein and saturated fat. They also occur in our bodies when we eat too much sugar and refined flour Dairy products are one of the most common causes of joint pain because they contain a protein that can irritate the tissues surrounding the joints.

Foods that reduce inflammation

Whole plant foods are naturally rich in anti-inflammatory compounds such as fiber, water and antioxidants and, of course, all the inflammatory compounds listed on the left are missing. The main anti-inflammatory products are yellow, red, orange and green leafy vegetables with a high content of carotenoids, such as spinach, cabbage and cabbage, nuts rich in monounsaturated fats such as almonds and walnuts, flax seeds or rich in chia in omega - 3, fruits such as strawberries rich in anthocyanins, blueberries, cherries and pineapples rich in bromelain, turmeric (because of curcumin) and ginger (because of the ginger compounds).

Slimming plants

Despite the dedication of counting calories, following the steps, going to the gym and the diets that eliminate everything we love or add a "miraculous" supplement, our society is increasingly affected by obesity and the diseases it derives from. A poor diet is not an effective long-term strategy and calorie restriction slows down the metabolism, which makes weight loss difficult.

Thinking about food in terms of nutritional density and calories is an easier and more effective way to combat weight loss. To lose weight, increase your portion of nutrient-rich foods and reduce your portion of junk food. The magic of this approach is that it changes the focus on creating positive health for you by consuming more delicious and satisfying things.

Nutrient-rich foods contain a large amount of vitamins, minerals and antioxidants. Vegetables, fruits, whole grains, beans, herbs and spices are nutrient-dense foods. Calorie-rich foods have a large amount of calories in relation to their volume Some examples are oils, sugars, dairy products, eggs, blue fish, meat and fried foods.

There are many foods rich in nutrients and calories, such as nuts, seeds and avocados. You want to eat these products because they have important minerals and other nutrients and small quantities can help you feel saturated. You should only eat them in smaller portions than other nutrient-rich foods.

Some foods do not contain nutrients even though they add calories per day. These are called empty calories. Allow your body to keep craving nutrients, even if you've added calories to your day. Examples are white rice, white bread, refined oils and refined sugar.

Having plants and focusing on choosing all foods rather than elaborate or refined versions increases nutrient density by reducing calorie density. It will also increase the consumption of water and fiber, increasing metabolism and improving digestion.

All the elements of the diet work together to satisfy and nourish the body at a deep level, thanks to which it develops, losing weight naturally. Over time, you will find that these intense cravings for bad food disappear simply because you feel that energy and health are building up. Add and develop, don't deny it or delete it, so you feel rich, happy and happy.

SNEAKY TIP TO LOSE WEIGHT WITHOUT PRIVACY

Use bowls and small dishes In a large plate or bowl, most people will take larger portions just too visually fill the space. For all meals, use dishes and bowls of the same size so that you know how to fill them with portions that will feed your day without going overboard.

Use only two or three flavors Our taste buds and the brain process our sensation of different flavors in a meal and we want to experience a certain amount of them before feeling satisfied. If we have too many different dishes and flavors at the same time, we generally eat more than necessary to have a good taste for each. An example of this manual is. So if we prepare a meal with only two or three different dishes, we will be satisfied before the filling is complete.

Eat with chopsticks It slows down (most of us) and generates small bites, which gives us a better chance to feel the signs of satiety in our body before eating too much.

Swallow between each bite It's more difficult than it looks! Try to check if you will be more aware of chewing. It also slows him down a bit to allow him to recover signs of satiety.

Brush your teeth between meals This is an excellent idea for oral hygiene and also reduces the likelihood of accidentally eating between meals. Scheduled snacks for fuel and nutrients are obviously a good idea, but it is best to minimize unnecessary bites.

Change the calorie density of food When cooking brown rice with another glass of water, the calorie density decreases .It will be the same, all you have to do is cook it a little. You can also do it with morning porridge to get more hydration to start the day; In addition, it is easier to digest.

Dilute the juice or soda One of the most effective ways to lose a few pounds with a shift is to replace juice or soda with water. You can drink lots of sugar, even 100% natural fruit juice, without realizing how many calories you've added to your day. Can't you go to a cold cup? Start by diluting drinks with water or sodas. Cutting them in half reduces sugar consumption in half. You can gradually try to dilute more until you just need a little taste in sparkling water or gas.

Plants and other benefits

There are many other potential health benefits when eating several plants. Here are some that people have found when switching to a plant-based diet.

The increases in **energy** exchange for nutrient-rich plant foods that provide energy levels, away from refined sugars and cereals, which blood sugar and inevitably increase many people are discovering that.

Facial cleansing: dairy products are one of the most common and clearly related triggers for acne. Sugar is also a common trigger, so when you cut down on refined sugars and switch to whole-grain sweets, your skin is likely to be cleansed.

Increased immunity The nutrients your immune system needs are rich in plants .Focus on dark green, red and orange fruits and vegetables and zinc seeds.

Better digestion With the great growth of fiber, many people have claimed that their digestion improves. Many of my client turtles felt that their pants fit better simply because they have less abdomen.

It calms the stomach too much meat, dairy products, processed and fatty foods, little chewing and stressed can cause the operation is either magician and guilty of heartburn and indigestion.

Faster recovery after training Athletes, runners and bodybuilders who use the percentage of plant diet that regenerate's quickly after training,

The end result: if you can be healthy and adequately fed with a plant-based diet, reduce the risk of debilitating degenerative diseases, help the planet, animals and people affected by animal husbandry, as well as eat interesting and different foods that have an amazing taste : What is still a reason not to make changes?

Would meals be as good as the ones I'm used to?

I can assure you that the plant-based diet is not limited to the plant diet (although leafy vegetables are quite important) The truth is that many times the same vegetables cannot supply enough for greater capacity .

It's a combination of

- Fruits such as apples, bananas, strawberries, oranges, berries, etc It is also your favorite fruit.
- Vegetables such as carrots, lettuce, cabbage, broccoli, cabbage, you can also add the vegetables you want to this list .
- Whole grains such as barley, millet, oats, wheat, quinoa, etc.
- Legumes such as lentils, chickpeas, black beans, etc
- Tubers such as potatoes, corn, peas and others, to name a few, which can become excellent and delicious delicacies .

You will be surprised by the variety of tasty dishes, delicious desserts and even healthy snacks that you can still eat following this lifestyle. So, I can say that your meals wouldn't be boring or boring, even if you have to give up on some of your favorite dishes and snacks.

Most of the time, your dish will focus on starchy foods that depended on it and that have been passed on to it for different generations .

Think about creating products like black beans, corn, peas, potatoes, brown rice, quinoa, beans and even chickpeas .They would have been prepared differently, but most of these dishes will be what you know and you can try them on the dishes you are used to Eat only .Sweet potato lasagna, mashed potatoes and salsa, black beans and rice burrito, which you can eat as much as you want with whole fruit

Talking about food all you want is another advantage of plantbased foods, you don't have to worry about counting calories or controlling the portion .Vegetable diets have a large volume that contains more fiber and water and this volume takes up more space, so it fills the stomach and deactivates the signs of hunger, even if you have consumed fewer calories than a normal hamburger.

Some people who follow this diet sometimes worry about eating some kind of green vegetables for calcium, beans for proteins, nuts for fats; etc.You should abandon this type of mentality, because the key point of this lifestyle is the choice of complete plant foods that you like best.

In the short term, you will not miss comfortable dishes such as hamburgers, French fries or fast food.

Would you be able to maintain this lifestyle?

Yes yes and yes!!! It will always be and will continue to be my answer to this question.

Experts agree that reducing refined processed and refined food products, such as í like eating your own food, order your favorite foods and replacing them with the help of herbs is good for the body.

After starting a plant-based diet, you will see first-hand results like lowering blood pressure and cholesterol, lowering medications, being able to adapt to old clothes and even discovering that it is better to sleep at night and wake up refreshed in the morning. Come on!

However, are you wondering how to motivate yourself to continue? If the results you see are not enough for you and you feel that you are starting to reach obstacles, know that you have many ways to navigate and switch to a healthy lifestyle.

You can achieve this lifestyle in several ways, some of which are;

1.   First, be your motivator

If you wish, you can continue with this lifestyle as an animator and encourage yourself by giving yourself the goals you intend to achieve .Set the records for yourself and work to break them For example, suppose you want to run with the dog at a distance and not be out of breath, or in a marathon, wear old clothes or have a certain size of dress .Record your progress in a written and award-winning newspaper or film I could also write notes which I could then read to encourage him and tell him how he was.

2.   Let others inspire you

If your success story isn't enough, let someone be your inspiration Videos of people on a plant-based diet talking about their success can also help you stay focused and remember that you've decided to do it.

Seeing how it works for others can help you stay on track and motivated .

3.   Never stop learning

Read books (like this one) on how to make healthy diets, natural cookbook guides, expert guides or nutrition books that can also be inspirational. Learning something new about this lifestyle can help you take the next step in the right direction and even give you advice on what you're doing wrong or right, and also how to do it better Reading will give you stimulating control that will help you stay on track.

4.   Be creative

Sometimes, just eating can be your biggest motivator Find a way to create your wishes using the shopping list or what you have in the refrigerator and you will find that following a plant-based diet is not difficult, and guess what? This way you will get some results, pride and satisfaction (I have a recipe chapter in this book, so keep reading).

5.   Use the online support group

Always remember that you are not alone in this, someone else has survived what you feel and survive. Even if your friends and family don't support you, there are hundreds of online groups dedicated to this lifestyle where their members share stories, fights, recipes and articles that can help you a lot.

Remember that at the beginning you can fall out of the car, but do not stay out of the car, suck it up and come back .

Is a vegetable diet expensive?

Did you know you can eat a diet rich in vegetables and all foods for around $ 3 a day? Yes, you read it correctly I'm not talking about every daily meal; I am talking about food **FOR THE DAY,** which is comparable to other meals .This is much less than spending on food, whether cooked at home or away from home.

Not only does he have control over the quality of the food he eats, he also eats tastier and healthier meals and also spends about a third of what he would have initially spent on his meals.

Herbal diet

Planning nutritionally balanced plant foods is not as difficult as it seems. It is known that some essential nutrients are linked to animal feed, such as protein and iron, and lack of knowledge of plant foods that can provide or dissuade some people from changing your diet.

If you eat a variety of healthy plant products, you will get most of the nutrients you need to be completely healthy, including proteins, vitamins and minerals such as iron and calcium. The only nutrients missing from plant foods are vitamin D and vitamin B $_{12,}$ which can be easily obtained from supplements.

It takes a little awareness and knowledge to start a healthy vegetable diet, but once you learn the basics, you can quickly and easily prepare healthy and balanced meals every day. Feel this wonderful feeling of strength when you understand how to eat properly and how to listen to your body's comments.

In the first chapter, we examine the key role that plants play in maintaining health and weight Now let's take a look at what a vegetable diet looks like.

What is this?

First, let's examine exactly what each term means.

Vegetarians do not eat animal meat (beef, fish, poultry, pork, lamb, etc) and cannot use products associated with the death of animals (such as skin).

Vegans do not eat products of animal origin (vegetarian diet, with the exception of dairy products, eggs, jellies or honey) and do not use products that cause death, cruelty or suffering of animals (such as skin, wool or other existing products that have been tested on animals) as far as possible and practical.

The supporters of products **made from** plants focus on whole plants and healthy lifestyle, avoiding highly processed foods and refined and highly processed oils and care for refined AZ.

Pescatarianseat fish but have no other animal meat Many eat dairy products or eggs.

Flexitarians eat mainly vegetarians, but are flexible in social situations.

The fact that motivation is primarily related to the environment, ethics or health can determine the choices that each person makes regarding what they buy and eat. Personally, I'm vegan.I am motivated by three motivating factors of vegan trifecta and I focus on whole foods.

However, the most important thing to look for and focus on how to enjoy a wide range of nutrient-rich foods and eat a large part of the diet, such as fresh fruits and vegetables .And it can make all this flavor phenomenal, so you'll never lose it.

DO NOT STORE THE TASTE

Some people think that a plant-based diet is about eating salads and not eating for the rest of their lives .If you are afraid or guilty of following a diet based solely on personal health, it is very difficult to maintain it in the long term, especially if eating is boring. Many customers come to me after trying to use plants, but they are so bored with food that they need help to maintain long-term balance.

Although I don't consider oils and sugars to be healthy foods, there is a general advantage to using them wisely to improve flavor and encourage long-term use of a healthy diet If a pinch of salt makes people eat with more carrots, if the bank produces oil, they want people to eat with more pumpkin treated as a state of victory It is a pity that. I would like so much attention after health and lack of flavor in bed, as they can work very well together Furthermore, the motivation to improve their health can go hand in hand with improving the health of our planet and reducing the suffering of animals .It turns out that trifecta can help you further strengthen your motivation, so it really becomes a lifestyle, not a diet Herbal groups.

At first glance, people often assume that the plant-based diet is extreme and restrictive .The truth is that now as a wider range of products that are read in the desired foods vegetables, fruits, seeds and spices, which I had never heard of, and cooking and eating is much more fun! I never feel limited or private; rather launched into a new exciting and tasty world full of options. Let me introduce you to the abundant world of plant foods to discover.

Vegetables are a starting point; They are so important that they should make up the bulk of your diet. They include all the leaves, roots, bulbs, stems, vines and flowers listed here Vegetables can be eaten in large quantities because most of them are water and fiber .They are full of vitamins and minerals and are an important source of potassium. Potassium is a mineral in the correct proportionsodium, works to regulate blood pressure Getting enough potassium is as important for people with hypertension as reducing sodium intake.

Foliage

Green leafy vegetables are one of the richest nutrients you can eat They contain many vitamins (especially K, A, C and folic acid) and minerals (such as iron, magnesium and potassium), as well as a large amount of chlorophyll, which cleanses the human system, especially the liver .If you feel tired of salads, try adding vegetables to a fruit cocktail or soup The vegetable puree is significantly reduced A wide range of leaves includes lettuce, cabbage, spinach, cabbage, chard, mizuna, rocket, Chinese cabbage, green cabbage, mustard, dandelion, escarole, watercress, sorrel and tatsoi.

Roots

Root vegetables are generally composed of complex carbohydrates and starch .Therefore, they are usually cooked before eating, because cooking breaks down the starch particles into easier to digest .However, carrots and radishes are widely consumed raw in North America Many tubers include carrots, beets, parsnips, kohlrabi, turnips, sweet potatoes, celery and radishes Many tubers, such as beets, radishes and turnips, also have very tasty leaves.

Light bulbs

This group includes onions, leeks and garlic The affirmation of garlic's reputation influences cardiovascular health; Many studies have shown that it reduces cholesterol, inhibits platelet aggregation (when platelets bind, forming blood clots) and lowers blood pressure Onions are also recommendedcardiovascular health because they have sulfur compounds similar to those that make garlic so strong.

Stems

Stem vegetables include asparagus, celery and kohlrabi All of them are very nutritious green vegetables with very few calories Kohlrabi is a relative of cabbage and broccoli, so it contains strong anti-inflammatory and anti-cancer compounds from this family of vegetables.

Lives

Although some of these vegetables are considered botanically fruit when it comes to nutrition and cooking, they fall into the category of vegetables .These vegetables have a high water content and are significantly reduced when cooked Since this category includes several vegetables, they have very different nutritional profiles, but vine vegetables are generally rich in carotenoids and vitamin C Vine vegetables include zucchini, squash, aubergines, cucumbers, peas, tuck, tomato and pepper

Flowers

Yes, flowers can also be vegetables! This group includes broccoli, cauliflower and artichokes Broccoli, like a dark green vegetable, is rich in nutrients and antioxidants. Although cauliflower has no color, it has similar nutrients and is as good for you as broccoli

Mushrooms

Mushrooms are not actually plants (they are mushrooms), but in nutritional terms they combine with vegetables The difference with mushrooms is that they eat organic matter and don't use photosynthesis like plants Since they are an organism completely different from other vegetables, they have a value in our diet, as they provide various nutrients such as selenium and copper, as well as strong anti-inflammatory compounds, protect against heart disease, protect from cancer and support the immune system Mushrooms are rich in minerals and protein calories and are also a good source of B vitamins.

Some mushrooms that can be found in local markets include chanterelles, shiitake, oysters, cremini, buttons, beehives and balloons .There are also many other types of edible mushrooms, including mushrooms used in Chinese medicine because of their medicinal properties, some of which are strong enough to fight cancer.

Fruit

Like vegetables, fruit also has a high content of water and fiber and many vitamins and minerals Fruits are an important source of rapid energy because they are digested and used by your body, the fastest of all food groups. Fruit contains concentrated antioxidants and, because they are sweet, they are often more pleasant than vegetables, especially for children.

The fruit of the tree is available in summer and autumn and includes apples, pears, plums and peaches Citrus fruits are best in winter and include oranges, grapefruits, lemons and limes Pure citrus juice can be used to flavor many plant-based recipes, including those that use vegetables Summer fruits include berries, grapes and melon Tropical fruits include bananas, pineapples, mangoes and kiwis.

Walnuts and seeds

Nuts and seeds are an excellent source of concentrated nutrients, especially minerals, and contain healthy fats that help the body absorb and use these minerals completely Studies have consistently shown that people who eat nuts have a lower risk of cardiovascular disease than those who don't eat nuts It is good to have many different types of nuts and seeds, because they all have different nutrients Almonds, walnuts, pistachios, cashews, walnuts, pumpkin seeds, sesame and flax seeds are popular.

Vegetable

Legumes are plants that bear fruit in pods; We usually eat fruit or seeds They are an important source of the amino acid lysine, are rich in fiber, vitamins and minerals and have low fat They are a healthier protein than animal products, as well as a cheaper protein per gram of protein. The most famous legumes are peas, beans, lentils, peanuts and alfalfa.

Whole grains

Whole grains contain complex carbohydrates to maintain energy and are a source of fiber, proteins, vitamins (especially vitamins B and vitamin E), minerals, essential fatty acids and antioxidants They are very difficult to digest raw, so they are usually cooked Some have hard outer shells, while others have a shell with a soft grain inside Always choose whole grains that have all their nutrients intact, rather than white, refined or polished beans that remain only in the starch cells .A wide range of whole grains with different textures and flavors is currently available These include rice, millet, buckwheat, oats, quinoa, spelled, barley and amaranth.

Spices and Herbs

Spices and herbs are not only a way to add rich flavor to dishes, but they also contain small amounts of important nutrients. A study conducted on vegetarian men who followed the Indian diet showed that they obtained from 39 to 79% of the essential amino acids they needed, together with about 6% of calcium and 4% of iron, only for spices in food.

Many spices contain protein and although they have too many grams, are a source of certain amino acids which may have a low content of plant foods Popular spices that will add flavor to the world include cumin, coriander, cinnamon, paprika and nutmeg.

Herbs such as parsley, coriander, mint, ginger and basil contain many nutrients and are more beneficial and tasty when eaten fresh Parsley gives women 22% of their daily recommendations on vitamin C and men 27% in just 4 tablespoons. All fresh herbs, such as green leafy vegetables, have a high content of antioxidants and chlorophyll, providing energy and helping the body neutralize free radicals.

Nutrients in the plant diet

Foods are made up of a mixture of macroelements (carbohydrates, fats and proteins) and microelements (vitamins and minerals) .The biggest component of your daily intake should be carbohydrates .Fat is the next largest section, followed by protein Since fats provide a dual-energy for the same volume, by observing the size of portions, fats and proteins should be nearly equal.

Most people should try to consume 60-70% carbohydrates, 2030% fat and 10-15% protein in the diet and up to 20% protein for athletes d ' is lite. If your energy consumption is about 1,500 calories, which I think is the average of my clients, which is between 225 and 263 grams of carbs, 33-50 grams of fat and 3856 grams of protein a day .The specific percentage that's right for you may be at the beginning or end of these ranges, but the ranges are appropriate for about 98 percent of the population .Your position may vary slightly during your life and seasons, so listen to your body. Despite some popular diet guides, it is unlikely that you will leave these ranges without any benefit Even older bodybuilders have never needed more than 20% protein and can actually be harmful to the kidneys and metabolism in general

However, if you're similar to most people, don't treat your foods like carbohydrates or fats, but like rice or avocado The advantage of plant foods is that they are much more balanced from a nutritional point of view than foods of animal origin, making it easier to stay within the normal ranges mentioned above without having to carefully follow what you eat .Let's take a look at the proportions of macronutrients in whole plant foods.

Carbohydrates

Some people worry about consuming too many carbohydrates when eating plant foods Carbohydrates are the main source of energy for the body and are completely healthy when consumed in the form of whole foods (such as whole grains, vegetables and fruit) because they contain many vitamins, minerals, antioxidants, water and fiber. Fiber is also a carbohydrate, but its function is to facilitate digestion rather than provide energy.

Whole grains and fruits have the highest carbohydrate levels, with a carbohydrate content of 70 to 90 percent. Eating a banana is a boost of instant energy. The best sources of fiber in the diet are psyllium or flax seeds and green leafy vegetables.

Protein

It is not as difficult as people think to get enough protein from plant foods .All plant foods contain some protein If enough calories consumed by a varied and balanced diet and regularly are legumes, protein you should consume more than enough and all essential amino acids (which are the building blocks of proteins) It is not necessary to combine multiple dishes in one meal to get all the necessary amino acids, which is a common mistake If you eat different products within 48 hours, the amino acids combine to do the job.

Legumes, including beans, have the highest total protein content in plant foods, about 18 to 25 percent; They are also important in vegetable diets because they provide enough lysine amino acid. The green leafy vegetables have a high percentage of protein of 40 percent, spices add a small but significant amounts of amino acids and whole grains add a good amount of protein in a balanced diet generally from 8 to 12 percent.

Fat

Your body needs enough fat in the diet to function, maintain metabolism, absorb and use minerals and some vitamins People with cold feet and hands, amenorrhea (loss of menstruation) or dry skin, hair or throat may need more fat in their diet, especially saturated fat such as coconut oil To be clear, eating healthy fats in reasonable quantities does not cause obesity.

Whole plant foods are the best source of healthy fats: avocado, nuts and seeds (including peanut butter and seeds) On average, about 80% fat .Whole grains and beans also have healthy fats and even fruit, vegetables, spices and almost all foods are even small For example, oatmeal flakes contain 15% fat.

Oils are 100% fat and you don't necessarily have to eat them, but they are excellent for a rich taste and full flavor on your plate, especially when you follow a healthier diet If you use oils, it is best to keep them to a minimum and use unrefined oils such as olives, coconut, sesame and avocado (Refined oils include rapeseed oil, soybean, sunflower and corn) You can easily skip vegetables for two with a teaspoon of oil.

However, this does not mean that you should never eat oils and some people could benefit from concentrated fats For example, flaxseed oil or concentrated DHA may be necessary for people with digestive problems and the use of omega-3 fatty acids.

THE DIFFERENCE BETWEEN A VEGETABLE DIET AND A VEGAN

DIET

This time I was training new students on the difference between a plant-based diet and a vegan diet I started by saying "if you think vegetable and vegan diets are the same, raise your hand" It happened as I thought: 90 percent of the class raised their hand.

Vegetable and vegan diets are really different Like a plant-based diet, it is a lifestyle, as is veganism.

The vegan diet seriously rejects all forms of animal products, such as eggs, birds, honey, dairy products and even eyebrows on animals used for clothing .Vegans are against scratched skin or pet clothing, skin or the use of animals to test products You may have noticed that some protests in fashion shows.

The vegetable diet aims to ensure that the food consumed is healthy, nutritious and beneficial for the body. It requires a lot of discipline and this diet provides plant substitutes for almost anything you can imagine in any animal food.

Everything you eat on a plant-based diet is intentional for healthy foods Up to 90% of Americans do not receive the recommended daily intake of fruit and vegetables; If you decide to follow a plant-based diet, you can be sure of getting all the necessary and balanced nutritional nutrients that your body deserves.

Diets are similar, but plant foods are consumed more protein plants and vegetables, this will reduce a animal products (or will remove a completely for some people) .There are people who follow a plant-based diet that consumes meat and there are people who follow or use animal products.

A vegan diet, especially if you think carefully, can be healthy, but plant-based diet has more benefits than a vegan diet because the diet is based on avoiding fully processed food plants and respecting all foods .They are densely nutritious depending on the description of it on all vegans; A good example are vegan cookies or vegan ice cream.

Thanks to the plant-based diet, it reduces the risk of heart disease and other types of diseases .This is one of the best ways to strengthen the immune system by supporting the body's metabolism. It is also a great way to start a weight loss journey.

Plant - diet-based is also known as whole or plant-based foods, it is as simple as it seems .It is a diet that has been developed based on the creation or without meals according to all foods (for example, natural foods that are whole, unrefined or minimally refined) and of vegetable origin (food grown on the farm or derived from plants) .

Right now, devotion, which I can say is simply changing your eating habits and lifestyle, eating refined, processed and stored food when you grow food on farms or derived from plants and some animal products (in some cases).

Herbal meals consist of

Vegetables: such as lettuce, cabbage, chard, pepper, peas, corn, etc.
Cereals: millet, quinoa, barley, rice, wheat, oats, etc.
Tubers: sweet potatoes, potatoes, sweet potatoes, carrots, beets, etc.
Legumes: beans, chickpeas, cannellini beans, lentils, black beans, etc.
Seeds: such as sorghum, chia seeds, sesame seeds, etc.
Fruits: such as apples, bananas, figs, grapes, strawberries, oranges, etc.

For many people who do not have a different understanding of what a food or vegetable lifestyle is, it seems or seems to think so;

Vegan diet: it is a completely vegetable diet that excludes meat, fish, dairy products and eggs .In principle, it excludes all forms of food of animal origin or derived animals.

Vegetarian diet: this is also a plant-based diet, but animal products such as a diary and eggs are included in meal planning .

Flexographic diet: it is a vegetarian diet that allows meat and fish, but it is still a vegetable diet .

Fish based diet: this is also a vegetable based diet which includes eggs, diary, fish and shellfish, but meat and poultry are excluded.

Plant-based diets are sometimes confused with a vegetarian or vegan diet, simply because this diet does not completely eliminate animal products, while a vegetarian or vegan diet does This diet simply selects multiple foods from plant sources.

It mainly depends on vegetables, fruits, seeds, legumes, nuts and whole grains because they make up the majority of their meals.

Although there are several types of plant diets and all claim to be associated with heart benefits (such as whole grains, fruits, vegetables, legumes, nuts and healthy oils) rich in fiber, vitamins and minerals that lower blood pressure and LDL, the risk of diabetes, helps maintain a healthy weight, you should still consider the types of plant foods and their sources.

A healthy vegetable meal should consist of appropriate portions of vegetables, whole grains, fruits, and proteins, healthy and healthy oils.

A plant-based diet or lifestyle is fairly easy and flexible because it consumes more plants, even if animal products are not fully available .

10 VEGETABLE SURVEILLANCE

There are so many trendy meals circulating in the news of the day They are fun because they are new and exotic .What might surprise you is the fact that many of the products you see every day are full of food nutrients .We give these daily superheroes the recognition they deserve.

1. Parsley

• High iron content that the body uses to produce energy and transport oxygen.

• Rich in vitamin C, which stimulates the immune system and promotes the absorption of iron.

• Extremely rich in vitamin K, which is part of a healthy bone structure, prevents blood clots and keeps nails strong.

• Rich in vitamin A, which maintains the correct functioning of the eyes, maintains the immune system and purifies acne, eczema and psoriasis.

2. Chia seeds

• One of the best sources of omega-3 fatty acids.

• Have a mixture of soluble and insoluble fiber to maintain a healthy intestinal function.

• Rich in calcium, which helps keep bones strong, minimizes muscle spasms and helps sleep.

3. Quinoa, amaranth and teff

- Rich in protein, a good alternative to beans if they give you gas.

- Higher levels of quercetin and kaempferol than other foods, both compounds that help reduce the inflammatory response to allergens.

- A good source of manganese (which supports the health of bones, skin and blood sugar), magnesium, folic acid (which helps maintain a healthy brain, cardiovascular system and pregnancy), zinc and vitamin E.

4. Buckwheat

- A good routine source, a plant pigment that can prevent blood clots, thyroid problems, memory loss, osteoarthritis and varicose veins.

- High content of B vitamins for energy and fat metabolism.

- High levels of antioxidants that fight free radicals that cause signs of aging, cancer, atherosclerosis and other problems.

- Contains a compound called D-chiro-inositol which helps balance blood sugar.

5. Berries

- An extremely rich source of antioxidants (which become organic or wild in the event of an overdose) that prevents cell damage and those found in the berries are particularly useful for maintaining memory.

- Low glycemic index (40-50; less than 50 means low), as shown in studies that improve blood sugar regulation.

- High manganese content, which helps maintain bone and skin health and balances blood sugar.

- Some women swear to help reduce hot flashes.

6. Squash

- Rich in vitamin A, which supports the health of the eyes, skin and immune system.

- High content of all carotenoids (plant pigments responsible for bright red, yellow and orange), including alpha, beta, lutein, zeaxanthin and beta-cryptoxanthin, which are antioxidants and have anti-inflammatory and immunological properties.

- The starch comes from polysaccharides which contain special compounds called homogalacturonan which have antioxidant, anti-inflammatory, antidiabetic and insulin regulating properties.

7. Avocados

- High potassium content to balance sodium for healthy blood pressure.

- Contains healthy fats that help the body absorb vitamins A, D and E, K and minerals Avocado fat is mainly monounsaturated, which has been shown to reduce heart disease risk, lower LDL cholesterol (bad type) and reduce oxidative stress in the blood.

- A good source of vitamins B, vitamin A and vitamin K.

8. Chickpeas

-

- High content of manganese, folic acid, iron and zinc. Complex carbohydrates for energy, as well as a protein source that helps muscles, digestion, hormones, neurotransmitters, genomes, blood pressure, energy and detoxification.

- It has a specific type of fiber that causes better regulation of blood fat, reduction of LDL cholesterol, total cholesterol, triglycerides, glycaemia and insulin secretion and is metabolized by bacteria in the colon to produce compounds that act as fuel for cells intestinal wall lining, which reduces the risk of colorectal cancer.

9. Brazil nuts and sunflower seeds

- High zinc content which helps strengthen the immune system and maintain healthy skin and male reproductive organs.

- A good source of selenium that maintains the immune system, detoxifies the liver, supports thyroid function, prevents certain types of cancer and maintains healthy hair, skin and nails.

- Rich in vitamin E, which is an antioxidant that helps protect the cardiovascular system.

10 ginger

- Helps digestion, increases metabolism; It has an antiinflammatory and immunostimulating effect.

- Gingerols can inhibit the growth of colon cancer cells and cause cell death in ovarian cancer cells.

- **Nutritional guidelines to stay strong and focused**

As a holistic nutritionist, I think you should move forward in a healthy lifestyle if you want to thrive and find the energy and health you are looking for .This path includes what you eat, what you don't eat, what you do during the day and, above all, the attitude you bring to the table.

But I don't think I have to do it all at once .And I definitely don't think you have to be perfect I am living proof, like the hundreds of clients. I have worked with, that a gradual, non-programmatic approach to diet change can work wonderfully. The main thing is to start .So focus on preparing dishes you like every day and celebrate your successes .Here are some tips and motivations to stay strong on this path.

Remove meat and seafood

Replace burgers with vegetarians Meat contains an inflammatory compound called arachidonic acid, along with saturated fat and cholesterol Cows produce 150 billion gallons of methane per day, which contributes significantly to global warming A pound of meat requires 2,500 liters of water.

Remove dairy products and eggs

Replace dairy products with almond milk and coconut yogurt and all other non-dairy products. Dairy products are one of the most common factors that cause food intolerance and a common cause of acne .The pound of cheese requires 900 liters of water A gallon of milk requires 1,000 liters of water.

Exchange the eggs with flax or chia seeds Or try Ceci Scramble in chapter 7 To produce a kilo of eggs, 477 liters of water are needed .While there is a debate about whether eggs are healthy, they don't add nutrients that we couldn't find elsewhere and for people with diabetes they can increase the risk of heart disease.

Avoid processed and refined foods

Processed foods are those whose shape has changed Every time we cook or pass, we process it .Man sauces butter í and beans are processed foods that are healthy because they still contain all its natural nutrients.

Refined products are those that have eliminated the parts, also eliminating the key parts of the diet White flour and white sugar are refined, as is white rice and oils such as rapeseed. When food is refined, they lose fiber, protein, vitamins and minerals. The part of the grain that remains after refining is mainly starch, with small quantities of some nutrients .That's why they are called empty calories .They allow your body to still crave nutrients, but add calories a day.

Focus on whole foods

All food is as close to its natural form as possible Fresh vegetables, fruits, whole grains, beans and legumes, as well as nuts and seeds are healthy products .By eating whole foods primarily, you maximize the nutrient density of all the vitamins, minerals and antioxidants in these products .It also reduces calorie density because these products contain a lot of fiber and water, so they fill you up without excess calories.

Chew your food

Not only does it slow you down a bit to enjoy a meal, but you can feel it more easily when it's full, but it's also the first important step in digestion without .Proper chewing of carbohydrates will not drop completely and may cause gas or indigestion later on

Avoid large portions

Portions in restaurants are usually much more of what you have to eat for a meal (unless you are in an elegant restaurant for the eyes) Contact the appropriate portions by trying the recipes and meals in this book .The recipes tell you how many portions you make .Take these numbers seriously, divide the dishes and see what it's like to eat a portion of regular size Chew slowly and start regulating the signs of hunger and satiety. This is the best way to find out how much you need to feed, but don't overfeed your body.

Good evening to eat

Most nutritional advice and healthy meals are boring .Have fun and make your taste buds happy by enjoying a fun meal .Yes, it can still be healthy. Try one of the pizza or vegetable burger recipes in this book or spend a Mexican evening with burritos, tacos or fajitas to prepare your dishes.

Take supplements

Vitamin B $_{12}$ supplements are needed when consuming a completely plant-based diet and for adults over the age of 50, regardless of the diet, as well as for people with digestive problems I.f anyone suggests eating eggs or other animal foods as a better or more natural way to get vitamin B $_{12}$, keep in mind that animals don't produce vitamin B $_{12}$; It is produced by bacteria in the digestive tract of animals. Older people and people with digestive problems cannot get vitamin B_{12} from feed, so supplements are the most effective way to get vitamin B_{12}.

The recommended daily allowance (RDA) in the United States for vitamin B $_{12}$ is 24 micrograms per day for most adults and 28 micrograms for pregnant or breastfeeding women. More recent research increases the ideal intake from 4 to 7 micrograms per day whyGroup B vitamins stimulate energy and the nervous system, it is better to take them in the morning and early afternoon so that they do not connect before bedtime.

Without vitamin D, you will not be able to properly absorb and use calcium and the lack of calcium and vitamin D will weaken your bones .Scientists are also starting to combine vitamin D deficiency with all types of health problems and diseases, including asthma and cancer .Carnivores should also be concerned here A 2009 study found that most vegetarians (59 percent) and those who eat meat (64 percent) do not have sufficient levels of vitamin D.

There is no vitamin D in plant foods, but our bodies naturally produce it when our skin is exposed to the sun .However, it is difficult to measure and trust because we produce different quantities depending on the color of the skin and other factors In winter, we generally don't have as much sun exposure as in summer .Further north, more winter will affect your vitamin D levels, and if it is really far north, you may not get it in winter The recommended daily dose is 600 IU per day, but for optimal health, supplementing between 1000 and 2000 IU per day has been shown to be a good level for most people Up to 4000 IU are safe for most adults.

The cause of calcium deficiency is not always a low intake and plant sources are often a better option than dairy products because they contain magnesium, which helps absorb the mineral However, because calcium is such a large nutrient, it is difficult to get enough food without consuming excessive calories .The average food intake is around 700 mg per day and the recommendation for adults is 1000 mg (up to 1,300 mg for the elderly). This means that a supplement that allows you to add these 300 mg more can be useful.

Our bodies also need two specific fatty acids from our diet: omega-3 and omega-6 Others can be made in our body if we usually eat enough fat .The tricky part is that our bodies need a certain proportion of omega-3 to omega-6 fatty acids Most food sources have too many omega-6 fatty acids, resulting in a relative deficiency of omega-3 fatty acids The strongest food sources for omega-3 fatty acids are ground flax, flaxseed oil, chia seeds and sachainchi oil and oil, which comes from an Amazonian tree Ground flax seeds are fantastic, but they can be difficult to digest and absorb If you want to make sure you have enough omega-3 fatty acids, oilsFlax, chia and sachainchi (also known as Inca nuts) are excellent ways to do this.

There is a specific type of omega-3 called DHA which is important for brain and nervous function Your body converts omega-3 to DHA, but it's not always efficient. Taking a 200 mg to 300 mg DHA supplement is often the best way to get this nutrient People who need more long-chain n-3 fatty acids, such as pregnant and lactating women, children and people with digestive or nervous problems, would benefit from DHA-rich supplements.

Digestive and / or probiotic enzyme supplements can be helpful to switch to a vegetable diet if your body has difficulty digesting beans Incomplete digestion is one of the main reasons for nutritional deficiencies, as well as food allergies and intolerances Probiotics are also needed after antibiotic treatment to populate a healthy intestinal flora.

FOOD COOKING PLANT

To be successful and take responsibility, you need to model the environment according to your goals, starting from what you bring into the kitchen and put on your body .If you make sure you have many healthy dishes in your kitchen, you can always prepare a balanced meal .Even if you don't have exactly what a specific recipe requires, you will need the ingredients you need to replace Let's change our kitchen.

Food storage

We throw flour, sugars and refined oils and choose healthy and unrefined versions Stock up on whole grains, beans and legumes and nuts.

• Whole grains (brown rice, quinoa, buckwheat, millet).

• Beans and legumes (chickpeas, beans, lentils).

• Walnuts (raisins, dates, dried apricots, berries).

• Unrefined oils (olives, coconut, toasted sesame seeds)

• Vinegars (apple, balsamic, wine).

• Whole wheat flour (whole wheat, spelled, oatmeal, buckwheat).

• Unrefined sweeteners (unrefined cane sugar, such as sucanate, coconut sugar, maple syrup, molasses, pure stevia).

• Sea salt.

• Spices (ginger, cumin, coriander, turmeric, pepper, cinnamon).

- Dried herbs (basil, oregano, thyme, dill, herbal blends).
- Food yeast.

Fridge

We throw meat, cheese, milk, eggs and packaged dishes Stock up on fresh produce, nuts and seeds and other dairy products.

- Green leaves (lettuce, cabbage, chard, spinach).
- Fresh herbs and spices (parsley, basil, mint, garlic, ginger).
- Green / starchy vegetables (cucumber, pepper, green beans, broccoli, mushrooms).
- Starchy vegetables (carrots, beets, sweet potatoes, winter squash)
- Onions (sweet, red, yellow, green).
- Fruit (apples, oranges, plums, grapes, melon).
- Nuts and seeds (almonds, walnuts, sunflower seeds, chia seeds, flax seeds).
- Peanut and seed butter (peanuts, almonds, cashews, sunflower)
- Non-dairy milk (almonds, soybeans).

Freezer

It's time to get rid of TV dinners, french fries, frozen waffles, ice cream, frozen cakes and desserts Stock up on fresh frozen products and homemade products.

- Frozen berries, mango, melon.

- Ripe frozen bananas for cocktails and cream sorbets.

- Frozen edamame beans, peas, corn, broccoli, spinach and other fresh frozen whole vegetables.

- Dishes that cook in large quantities and freeze them in individual portions (soups, stews, chilli, tomato sauce, vegetarian burgers)

- Healthy sweets (biscuits, cupcakes, biscuits, fruit cakes).

Fast food factory at home

Sometimes we don't have time to respect the rules .These days I have made a sketch of a balanced meal so you can combine it with what is in your kitchen.

Beater

Prepare the perfect nutritious cocktail to start the day and feed it You will need:

- Glass and straw: Drinking reusable straw minimizes contact with the teeth for better dental health and the use of an insulated cup or travel mug keeps the cocktail fresh in the morning.

- Creaminess: bananas (frozen IT brands, such as ice cream), avocado, peanut butter or milk without milk.

- Omega-3: 1 tablespoon of flaxseed or chia.

Protein: a handful of oatmeal or quinoa or a spoonful of vegetable protein powder.

- Fruit: about 1 cup of berries, melon, grapes, in the form of apples, whatever you want.

- Strengthen vegetables: vegetables such as spinach, sprouts or cabbage; vegetables such as cucumbers or carrots; Fresh herbs like mint or basil.

- Increased food levels: fresh ginger, powdered green leaves, matcha powder, probiotics, blueberries or goji powder, cocoa beans.

Bowl

Build the perfect bowl for lunch or dinner that will provide you with all the nutrients and fuel you need for the rest of the day You will need:

Bowl: Get a pair of the same size to keep portions consistent

- Green leafy vegetables: take a handful or two as much as you like, lettuce, rocket, spinach, cabbage, chard, parsley or other vegetables.

- Starchy vegetables and / or whole grains: about 1 cup of sweet potatoes, winter squash, brown rice, quinoa, spelled, soba noodles, rice noodles, etc.

- Beans or legumes: about ½ cup of chickpeas, black beans, lentils, edamame or other legumes.

- Other vegetables: about 1 cup of raw vegetables, such as cucumber, pepper, tomato and avocado; grilled, such as courgettes, aubergines and mushrooms; or steamed like broccoli, carrots and beets.

- Nuts or seeds: a small whole handful (pumpkin, cashews, almonds) or peanut butter, which can be used as a base for the sauce.

- Salsa: a long and generous drizzle Try the recipes in this book, such as sesame and baked miso sauce, green goddess sauce or creamy balsamic sauce or check the ingredients to see if you can find different foods in the shop.

DIET BASED ON HEALTHY PLANTS

We all know that plant-based diets are important for our wellbeing and health, especially when it comes to preventing heart disease .However, as Fred's father has experienced, scientists have discovered that there are plant-based diets that can be harmful to your heart's health.

According to the Center for Disease Control (CDC) in the United States, it has been discovered that over six hundred thousand people die of heart disease every year .The root cause of this death has been identified as poor nutrition, which is the driving force behind heart disease.

Numerous researches have been conducted to demonstrate the numerous benefits of whole grains, vegetables, legumes, flax seeds and fruit; These products have been identified as the right type of diet to stop coronary heart disease.

Another analysis has shown that diets are vegetables the best type of food desired for people and for ischemic heart disease .

According to the latest and complete study of the benefits and risks of the plant-based diet The study was conducted on approximately 209,289 people, consisting of 43,259 men and 166,030 women, according to the study of health nurses and the study of health professionals. The study continued for about 20 years to understand the lifestyle, health behaviors and medical history of the participants. Participants in this study never had a stroke, cancer, coronary heart disease or coronary artery surgery During follow-up, approximately 8,631 patients with ischemic heart disease.

One of the main reasons why these studies were conducted was the distinction between different diets: plant-based diet and vegetarian diet .He intended to distinguish between different types of foods derived from plants, taking into account the pros and cons.

Scientists decided to focus on diets and developed three different diets I'm:

A plant-based diet consisting of foods derived from unhealthy plants These include refined cereals, sweet drinks, candies and potato.

Plant foods that used the intake of plant foods and allowed foods containing animals or nutrients .

Herbal products that focus on healthy plant foods: whole grains, vegetables, fruit, legumes (these products are more organic).

NUTRITIONAL CULINARY GUIDE
FOR FOOD PLANTS

Buy fresh

Buy products in the coolest way possible, grown locally and organically whenever possible Grow yours if you can Sprouts and herbs can be easily grown on the windowsill If you are using whole grains and spices in your pantry, replace those old after about a year. If you start with fresh ingredients and high quality , your meals will naturally have a better flavor.

Choose the products you like

Most of the time, choose the vegetables and other products you like best Get diversity by launching a new one from time to time, but it doesn't always have to be this way .Some products are naturally tastier than others for most people. The natural sweetness of pumpkin, sweet potatoes, red peppers, carrots and beets makes them more attractive Vegetables and legumes are often also softer and sweeter than their fully developed counterparts.

Choose your cooking methods

Use the correct method for cooking vegetables .Avocados are better raw, broccoli is lightly prepared to perfection (but becomes bitter if overcooked), sweet potatoes and pumpkin are delicious in the oven or in the oven. The cooking of whole grains takes different times and can be cooked earlier to improve the taste.

Find good combinations

The combination of food on a plate consists of a combination of flavors (sweet, salty, sour) and textures (crunchy, soft) Color also plays an important role, making the vase visually more attractive Interested in combining opposites (bittersweet) or similarities (all green). It's also about personal preferences, so try the recipes as a reference, then play with the combinations to see what you like.

Use the salt

A small amount of salt does a lot to make the food delicious Softens the bitterness of vegetables and their consistency .It helps destroy the cell walls of plants, making them easier to digest production. It helps to combine all the flavors of the dish, so that the hummus does not know the individual ingredients, but the hummus .While cooking, use salt, rub it to moisten the vegetables before baking or sprinkle a lightly salted sauce in a bowl or salad.

Season your beans

Beans and beans don't taste good Make them more interesting as follows:

• To be combined with fresh and tasty fruit or vegetables.
• Add spices, herbs or tea to the water while cooking.

- Use part of the vegetable broth or juice as part or all the water for cooking.
- Season with spices and salty sauces.

Greet

Each dish can taste excellent with the right seasoning or sauce .Pickling vegetables in a good sauce will soften the bitterness and texture and help combine the flavors of the vegetables and sauce Marinate the beans and whole grains in sauce for an hour (or day) to saturate them, so that they are full of flavor.

Add dessert

Use some natural sweetness in your kitchen .Try a balsamic sauce, a maple syrup or an apple mousse; Add apples, oranges, dried cranberries or raisins to the salad or soup.

Use healthy fats

Fat makes the dish richer and more satisfying. Fat has the flavor of spices and herbs, so use it in a high flavor dish. Use more fat by following a plant-based diet or if you are not used to healthy cooking. For most foods, try using fats instead of fats, which are naturally part of cooked foods such as nuts, seeds and avocados The mixture of peanut butter and seeds or avocado are an excellent cream base for a sauce or salsa.

Camouflage

Be smart! Mix vegetables and greens in soups, sauces or cocktails Cook the vegetables in delicacies such as carrot cake, courgette bread, pumpkin muffins, chocolate cake with beet infusion and sweet potato biscuits.

LIVE FOOD PLANS

Are you ready to increase the nutritional value, taste and energy you get from food? Everything can happen immediately, I promise! I have compiled these meal plans to show you how to prepare delicious herbal dishes that provide balanced nutrition and nutrition for the day.

Plans set for the next three weeks eliminate the guesswork in the kitchen about the plant-based diet by offering three meals a day and snack options that you can choose from in weeks Chapter 3 contains more recipes than food plans. This leaves room for flexibility, so if something in your eating plan doesn't satisfy you, change it to another recipe.

These meal plans use leftovers to make your life easier, because most of us don't have time to prepare three meals a day .Breakfast and lunch must be brought and removed from Monday to Friday I will also give advice on how to prepare for the week so that you can prepare yourself for success.

Desserts are not included in the plan, but you can try desserts in Chapter 11 if you wish, or if you have a party or shared meal where you want to bring something you like.

Our goal is to feel healthy, full of energy, content and happy at the end of this plan.

Get some sleep

There are studies showing that sleep affects the part of the brain that controls willpower .So if you're awake, it's more difficult to resist temptation .Your ability to make clear decisions has decreased, which increases the likelihood of resorting to foods you don't really need.

It is also less able to handle stress constructively, making it more susceptible to overeating or other negative compensation mechanisms. Regular, high-quality sleep will not only make you healthier and more energetic, but will also help you control your desires. Here are some ways to cultivate healthy sleep habits

- Try to have approximately the same time to wake up and sleep every day
- Do not use the TV, computer, tablet or phone 30 minutes before bedtime
- Do not exercise after lunch
- Lack of caffeine after 2 p M
- After dinner without sugar
- Try meditation, recovery yoga or something relaxing at night

Active three times a week

Exercise is critical to maintaining bone mass, cardiovascular health, lymphatic and immune function and can help prevent diabetes .The exercise also releases hormones into the blood that make you feel happy, reduce hunger andIt usually maintains the proper functioning of the body .Try doing a quick workout after work and you may find that you don't need such a big meal for dinner.

Regular exercise helps reduce fatigue, depression, tension, worry and inappropriate feelings; Improve mood and ability to cope with stressful situations .When you get stronger and have more stamina, your body works more effectively Start with something you like: walking, skating, hula hula If you like it, you are much more likely to keep it long term .Indicate something you can do for 20-30 minutes, three times a week .It doesn't always have to be the same Mix to keep your curiosity When you get used to it, you can add more days, spend more time or try something more intense.

Don't stress that you're perfect

Stress affects health and excessive stress from eating is counterproductive .It would be nice if you could always eat the perfect diet and maintain an ideal exercise plan, but I don't know anyone who can do it every day of your life .Don't feel guilty if you have a day that isn't perfect, because it will only bring negative energy into your life. Some people eat more when they don't feel well I don't like using the words "slip", "trap" or "mistake" because .I believe that everything we do is only part of life and makes us the person we will be tomorrow.

Don't punish yourself with less food or more exercise Instead, take a letter every day and go further, revitalized, to maintain or eventually adapt your plan in the future so that it works for you in real life.

Listen to your body and enjoy!

Keeping balance doesn't always mean strict rules or eating plans; It means finding a balance for your body's needs .Now that you are looking for better health, you can get back in touch and trust your instincts to continue learning what works for you Eat consciously, chew your food well, enjoy the flavors and recognize when you've eaten enough.

When your body is balanced and adheres to the basic principles of long-term healthy eating, you should be able to listen to your body's messages about what needs to be healthy .Each person is different and will have a different way of being healthy .But your body's messages can be distorted or silenced when they are unbalanced, so at first it is difficult to determine whether what you feel is real desire or hunger.

Positive energy can have a big impact on achieving your goals It is unfortunate that many diet programs focus on avoiding unhealthy foods by switching to a healthy diet because it is much more fun and effective to focus on eating good foods Find some good foods that you really like, such as fruit, nuts or a special dinner and eat them often to feel happy and excited for a healthy lifestyle.

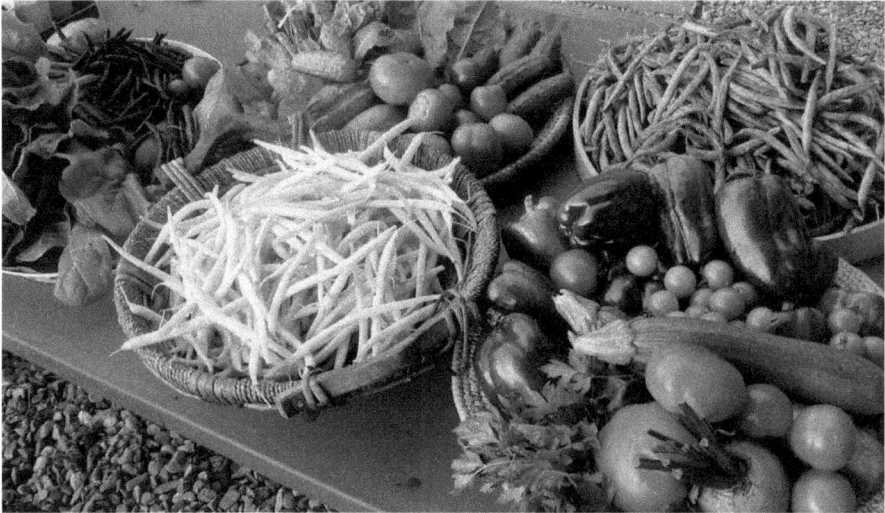

START A PLANET-BASED DIET

Statistics have shown that more and more people are choosing a plant-based diet; People are aware of the benefits of a plantbased diet. In the United States, over 1/3 of consumers actively consume more plant products.

Stars such as F1 champion Lewis Hamilton Will I Am, the awardwinning Hollywood director Ava DuVernay, the writer, Alicia Silverstone, the actress and musician Moby have also supported the cause of the plant-based diet .

Why do you have to follow a plant-based diet?

According to research and various studies, it is known that a plant diet also prevents and reverses type II diabetes, as well as advanced cardiovascular diseases .

Studies have also shown that people who use a plant-based diet are easier to maintain weight, reduce the risk of sudden death and reduce the risk of heart disease .

Doctors, nutritionists and health experts have linked the continuous consumption of a plant-based diet with the treatment and prevention of high (and bad) cholesterol, hypertension and reduced risk of certain types of cancer.

The Academy of Nutrition and Dietetics has found that properly planned vega, joint food, vegetarian diet, rock (this includes sleeping with the desired food, the kiro spirit, vegetables), as the desired diet is healthy , nutritionally dense and is the best for all people regardless of their age or age their lives such as childhood, adolescence, adulthood, pregnancy and old age Athletes can also choose this diet.

I'm sure you will be impressed by the benefits .I have mentioned and you will be happy to get on the train; Despite how big these points are, you should understand that the transition is a bit difficult Some people wanted to make the transition, but they couldn't keep up.

This means that your initial energy for the beginning must be strong enough to support you while living this lifestyle .It means a lot of planning, willpower and commitment.

I had to tell my clients to move gradually .If you are used to drinking soda and popcorn every day for the past 10 years, it may be almost impossible not to do it for a week.

These are some of the simple strategies that have helped me and helped my clients gradually and smoothly switch to the plantbased diet.

Start with small steps

Switching to a plant-based diet is no different than learning to walk after the leg has been in a cast for months. It is best to start with plant foods that you normally consume. It can be a burrito with beans and rice, oatmeal, three fried chillies, spring spaghetti, fried vegetables or lentil stew.

This way you can start gradually and develop these dishes .It is a better way to choose this diet because only human nature is engaged in what we love It is best to build up slowly because it relieves any pressure you may initially feel.

Reduce the consumption of processed foods and meat

Instead of cutting processed meat and food products, at the same time, you can begin to reduce the consumption of animal and processed products Change the aspect ratio from 80:20, 70:30, 60:40, 50:50, 45:55, 40:60, 30:70, 20:80, 10:90 to get a 100% diet in plants . The first series of numbers refers to processed foods, meat and products of animal origin, while the second series refers to foods of vegetable origin.

When you do it this way, it will give your mind and body time to adapt to this diet .You can start by adding a few tablespoons of salad to a meal, then replace the meat with vegetable substitutes such as Portobello or Bulgarian dried mushrooms.

Start with a healthy herbal breakfast

After starting the first two steps, you can continue with the third step, which is to have a vegetable breakfast every day Make this the first meal of the day so that your body warms up gradually After balancing it, you should go for lunch and then make this change for snacks and dinners

Check your protein intake

Although our bodies are in need of about one gram of protein per kilogram of body weight, many people take it every day to the amount a of a request.

The fact that the body needs protein not it a reason for its excessive consumption, as it can also be harmful to the body .You just have to find foods that can provide you with nine important amino acids that your body really needs.

The good thing is that foods obtained from healthy plants contain proteins and amino acids in various proportions .After consuming the right amount of calories the body needs, it will be easy to concentrate on whole foods .It also means that it will be difficult to have a protein deficiency.

You know what you consume

You need to know what you are doing and how to prepare perfect and healthy meals for you .There are many vegetable products that can be found on the market, such as cheeses and fake meats, but they are very elaborate. It can be very harmful to the body because it is very saturated with saturated fats, amino acids, flours, salts, refined oils and sugars.

Therefore, it is better to know what you are buying and read the label before buying Search and chooses organic and whole foods .Try reading about nutrition and what you eat. Discover different ways to prepare different dishes.

If you can hire a vegetable dietician, help him plan and choose the best food for him. I have had the opportunity to do it for people and this has facilitated the transition of my customers .This lifestyle can be difficult, but a dietician can make it easier.

You will never run out of healthy food

There are many healthy products that you can easily find by visiting supermarkets and shops .This will allow you to integrate plant products more easily and change your lifestyle. There is dairy-free milk, tofu, french fries and tempeh.

In addition, there is always something you can afford, regardless of cost, to take some 'time to switch to a vegetarian brokers and fresh, with products the next time you visit the supermarket He is never short of healthy and nutritious food based on plans; Keep some in your bag, drawers, workplace, refrigerator and work surface

Be creative about what you eat

Start eating around and find out how to make it work creatively .You can learn the recipes and try something new on your own; The more you try, the better you will be Discover new ways to prepare salads, soups and daily use so you don't get bored when the same thing is served every day.

Take snacks whenever you want (I'll show you how to prepare them in the following chapters) .Take some time to learn recipes from various blogs and restaurants.

Find a group
Social networks have made it easy to reach almost anyone or anything. Find groups that can help you learn and learn new

skills They can encourage you when you need it and teach you what to do when your desires begin; You can also ask questions.

In general, it should be perceived as a young child who is learning. This way you don't force yourself to learn .Find the right one for you and stay with him.

DIET PLAN

Week 1

	Breakfast	**lunch**	**Dinner**	**Ideas for snacks**
Mon day	Coffee machine of spinach and mushrooms	Puree of cauliflowe r and casserole of b eans green	Left on the lunc h Green milkshak e	Bathroom of Moon Blue
Tue sday	Cozy cabin panc akes	Burrito Bowl	Spaghetti with Mediterranean vegetables	Summer Chi ckpea Salad
We dne sday	Sunrise bruschetta with ricotta, sugar in powder and grat ed rind of lemon	Rice and black bea ns	Thai noodles	Bars cake ch eese with cru st of nut
Thu rsda y	Spicy Tofu Scrambled	Mixed vegetables Soup of spinach	Pineapple Papaya Fried Ri ce	Burning pop pers with to mato and chipotle sauc e
Frid ay	Avena cut in stee l of turmeric	Tagliatelle of courg ette with Portobello Bologne se	Burrito Bowl	Cake cheese chocolate wh ite petit fours
Satu rday	The big pumpkin bre ad with cream ch eese	Mixture of Achar	Sopa Mexicana De Lentils	Pie of apple r aw
Sun day	Spicy Tofu Scrambled	Spaghetti with Me diterranean vegeta bles	cabbages of Bru ssels	Cake of chee se and banan a

Week 2

	Breakfast	lunch	Dinner	Ideas for snacks
Monday	Cozy cabin pancakes	Rice and black beans	Thai noodles	Burning poppers with tomato and chipotle sauce
Tuesday	Spicy Tofu Scrambled	Spaghetti with Mediterranean vegetables	Puree of cauliflower and casserole of beans green	Cake of cheese and banana
Wednesday	Cupcakes with orange chai tea	Mixture of Achar	Sopa Mexicana De Lentils	Pie of apple raw
Thursday	Oatmeal with fruits and nuts	Burrito Bowl	Wholemeal macaroni with cottage cheese and cheddar cheese	Bars cake cheese with crust of nut
Friday	Gruel of protein	Cauliflower and tomato curry with coconut	Left on the lunch Herbal hummus	Guacamole Green Pea
Saturday	The Jumble cheesy for DIY	Sopa Mexicana De Lentils	Tagliatelle of courgette with Portobello Bolognese	seitan flares
Sunday	Tea of mint and thyme	Cauliflower and tomato curry with coconut	Pineapple Papaya Fried Rice	Churning of blueberry and avocado

Week 3

	Breakfast	lunch	Dinner	Ideas for snacks
Mon day	Capuchino vega n Cozy cabin panc akes	Cauliflower and tomato curry with coconut	Left on the l unch Green milks hake	Custard of frui ts
Tues day	The big pumpkin bre ad with cream c heese	Cauliflower and tomato curry with coconut	Walnut Taco s	Soup of beet si lver
Wed nesd ay	Budín of chia gr een	Thai noodles	Pineapple Papaya Frie d Rice	Summer Chic kpea Salad
Thur sday	The Queen Bloo dy Mary Mary	Chickpea Tacos Thai noodles	Garlic Hash Brown with Kale	Cake cheese c hocolate white petit fours
Frid ay	You have to frittata!	Delicious compote Burrito Bowl	Sopa Mexica na De Lentils	Pie of apple ra w
Satu rday	Avena cut in ste el of turmeric	Spaghetti with Medit erranean vegetables	Cauliflower and tomato curry with coconut	Burning popp ers with tomat o and chipotle sauce
Sun day	Millefeuille of m ushrooms and c heese	Puree of cauliflower and casserole of bea ns green	Vegetables i n escabeche	Salad of fruits to cream

TOP 50 DIETARY REGULATIONS BASED ON NUTRITIONAL SERVICES

We have been talking about what to eat for a long time, now is the time to work. Now you need to know how to do what's really good for you. It is the only way to be 100% sure of what you eat.

I will teach you how to prepare all foods for plants and what to do with vegetables, fruits, legumes, tubers, cereals and other whole foods .I'd give you recipes for all kinds of dishes from all over the world.

It doesn't matter if you are a beginner or a chef; I'm sure you will learn something new or something that can improve. At some point, I'm sure you will do wonders in your kitchen.

Recipes

In recipes, we use knowledge and have fun In the following chapters, I will give you more than 100 recipes to discover the flavors of plant foods and, I hope, help you fall in love with this lifestyle.

These recipes have zero cholesterol, low saturated fat content, balanced sodium-potassium, healthy heart and rich in antioxidants. Although they all have immune stimulating and anti-inflammatory properties, I will mention some recipes that are turbocharged in this area due to some specific ingredients I indicate which recipes are particularly suitable for children, without nuts, gluten and quick preparations (15 minutes or less)

There are many meals here besides those of the meal plans, along with delicious and nutritious desserts, so you can enjoy a longterm healthy meal.

Max Power Smoothie

It produces 3 to 4 cups of cups

Preparation time: 5 minutes

FAST PREPARATION GLUTEN FREE pleasant for children Anti-inflammatory immunity enhancer

It is a delicious breakfast base to start the day with optional supplements to maximize nutrient density .

The stems and the chard can be hard, so it is better to tear off the leaves of the stem and work only with the leaves Vegetables and carrots work best if you have a powerful blender like Blendtec or Vitamix .

If you have a regular mixer, skip the fresh vegetables and use a green powder like vegetables brand to receive an injection of nutrients without brittleness

- 1 banana
- ¼ cup oatmeal and 1 tablespoon protein powder plant
- 1 tablespoon of flax seeds or chia seeds
- 1 cup of raspberries or other berries
- 1 cup chopped mango (frozen or fresh)
- ½ cup of raw milk (optional)
- 1 cup of water
- BONUS DRIVERS (OPTIONAL)
- 2 tablespoons of fresh parsley or chopped basil

1 cup of chopped fresh cabbage, spinach, chard or other greenery
- 1 peeled carrot
- 1 tablespoon of grated fresh ginger

1 Slide everything into the blender until smooth, adding more water (or non-dairy milk) if necessary

2 Add some, some or all the necessary additional improvements Puree to mix

<u>Go ahead:</u> <u>buy more bananas so that when ripe they can be peeled and placed in the freezer. Frozen bananas ensure maximum creaminess of the cocktail</u>

Chai Chia Shake

It produces 3 desired cups

Preparation time: 5 minutes

GLUTEN-FREE PREPARATION WITH ANTIINFLAMMATORY WALNUT

Chai spices can aid digestion, improve blood sugar balance and increase metabolism .Chia seeds are a fantastic source of omega3 fatty acids, calcium, phosphorus and manganese .Prepare these delicious cocktails to enjoy your day trip as an alternative to the super nutritious chai latte.

- **1 banana**
- **½ cup of coconut milk**
- **1 cup of water**
- **1 cup of alfalfa sprouts (optional)**
- **1 to 2 soft Medjool dates, without bone**
- **1 tablespoon of chia seeds or heart of ground flax or hemp**
- **¼ teaspoon ground cinnamon**
- **A pinch of ground cardamom**
- **1 tablespoon of freshly grated ginger or 1/4 teaspoon of ground ginger**

Clean everything in the blender until smooth, adding more water (or coconut milk) if necessary.

<u>You know</u> <u>Although dates are very sweet, they don't cause high blood sugar levels They are excellent for increasing sweets, increasing the intake of fiber and potassium</u>
TropiKale Breeze

It produces 3 to 4 cups of cups

Preparation time: 5 minutes

FAST PREPARATION

GLUTEN FREE pleasant for children
Antiinflammatory immunity enhancer

Pineapple is a natural metabolism enhancer, it has an enzyme that helps digestion and helps reduce the bitterness of cabbage. If you've never tried vegetables in a cocktail, you should try it first .You can change the cabbage to spinach if you want to start a milder taste .We also use avocado to get creamy instead of bananas, making it a low carbohydrate option compared to other cocktails Add a teaspoon of matcha green tea powder to increase the dose if necessary.

+ **1 cup chopped pineapple (frozen or fresh)**
+ **1 cup chopped mango (frozen or fresh)**
+ **½ to 1 cup of chopped cabbage**
+ **½ avocado**
+ **½ cup of coconut milk**
+ **1 cup of water or coconut water**
+ **1 teaspoon matcha green tea powder (optional)**

Clean everything in the blender until smooth, adding more water (or coconut milk) if necessary.

Did you know that Matcha green tea powder contains catechins that minimize inflammation and maximize fat burning potential?
Hydration station

It produces 3 to 4 cups of cups

Preparation time: 5 minutes

QUICK REINFORCEMENT

WITHOUT FRIEND IMMUNITY FRIEND GLUTEN

If you are subject to morning headaches, this is a shock to you Headache is often a sign of dehydration, so increase your water and electrolyte intake with this strong and delicious smoothie .It is also ideal after training or a race to replenish and refresh.

- 1 banana
  1 orange, peeled and sliced or 1 cup of pure orange juice
- 1 cup of strawberries (frozen or fresh)
- 1 cup of chopped cucumber
- ½ cup of coconut water
- 1 cup of water
  ½ cup of ice

BONUS DRIVERS (OPTIONAL)

- 1 cup of chopped spinach
  ¼ cup of fresh mint, chopped

1 Put everything in the blender until smooth, adding more water if necessary

2 Add bonus updates if needed Puree to mix

<u>Advantage:</u> <u>Pour your cocktail into an insulated travel mug or thermos so that it stays cool while traveling</u>

Mango of Madness

It produces 3 to 4 cups of cups

Preparation time: 5 minutes

WITHOUT FRIEND IMMUNITY FRIEND GLUTEN FREE

Charge your immune system rich in vitamin C .The cocktail is also rich in beta carotene for sharp eyes and clean skin .If you don't have a high-powered blender or don't want a carrot in a cocktail, you can skip it.

- **1 banana**
- **1 cup chopped mango (frozen or fresh)**
- **1 cup chopped peach (frozen or fresh)**
- **1 cup of strawberries**
- **1 carrot, peeled and minced (optional)**
- **1 cup of water**

Rub everything in the blender until smooth, adding more water if necessary

Options: if you can't find frozen peaches and fresh peaches, it's not in season, use only mango or other strawberries or try melon

PB Milk Chocolate Smoothie

It produces 3 to 4 cups of cups Preparation time: 5 minutes

QUICK PREPARATION FOR CHILDREN

This cocktail is so delicious that you may not think it is healthy But this is 100% goodness. It covers all its nutrients to start the day well, keep it for dinner and is an excellent counterweight to the sadness of Monday morning.

+ **1 banana**
+ **¼ cup oatmeal and 1 tablespoon protein powder plant**
+ **1 tablespoon of flax seeds or chia seeds**
+ **1 tablespoon of bitter cocoa powder**
+ **1 tablespoon of peanut butter or almond butter or sunflower seeds**
+ **1 tablespoon of maple syrup (optional)**
+ **1 cup of alfalfa or chopped spinach (optional)**
+ **½ cup of raw milk (optional)**
+ **1 cup of water**

BONUS DRIVERS (OPTIONAL)
1 teaspoon of maca powder
1 teaspoon of cocoa beans

1 Slide everything into the blender until smooth, adding more water (or non-dairy milk) if necessary 2 Add bonus updates if needed Puree to mix

Did you know that the flavonols present in cocoa seem to help protect the mucous membrane of blood vessels and postmenopausal women seem to obtain the greatest cardiovascular benefits from cocoa consumption?

Pink panther smoothie

It produces 3 desired cups

Preparation time: 5 minutes

QUICK REINFORCEMENT WITHOUT RAPID IMPULSING PREPARATION THE IMMUNITY ANTIFLAMMATORY

This cocktail is silky smooth with little dynamics. Berries are a rich source of vitamin C and contain numerous unique nutrients that provide protective, antioxidant, anti-inflammatory and liver protection and prevent cancer (especially breast, colon, lung and prostate) and gastrointestinal infections uric.

- **1 cup of strawberries**
- **1 cup of chopped melon (any type)**
- **1 cup of blueberries or raspberries**
- **1 tablespoon of chia seeds**
- **½ cup of coconut milk or other non-dairy milk**
- **1 cup of water**

BONUS DRIVERS (OPTIONAL)

1 teaspoon goji berries

2 tablespoons chopped fresh mint Instruction:

1 Slide everything into the blender until smooth, adding more water (or coconut milk) if necessary 2 Add bonus updates if needed Puree to mix

<u>Options:</u> <u>If you don't have (or don't like) coconut, try using sunflower seeds to strengthen the resistance of zinc and selenium</u>

Banana and nut Smoothie

It produces 2 to 3 cups of cups Preparation
time: 5 minutes

GLUTEN FREE PREPARATION FOR CHILDREN

It is like banana bread in a glass Make a quick breakfast or dessert Almond butter is already creamy, but if you have a strong blender, it is also very tasty with 2 tablespoons of walnuts instead of almond butter .Make it super thick for a smoothie bowl covered with fruit muesli or muesli and slices of fresh fruit.

- 1 banana
- 1 tablespoon of almond butter or sunflower butter
- ¼ teaspoon ground cinnamon
- A pinch of ground nutmeg
- 1-2 tablespoons of dates or maple syrup
- 1 tablespoon of flaxseed or chia or hemp seeds
- ½ cup of raw milk (optional)
- 1 cup of water

Clean everything in the blender until smooth, adding more water (or non-dairy milk) if necessary.

Options: you can prepare a pumpkin spice cocktail by adding 1 cup of boiled pumpkin and a pinch of allspice

Oatmeal at night

Make 1 serving

Preparation time: 5 minutes / Cooking time: 5 minutes or overnight

GLUTEN FREE PREPARATION WITH NO FRIENDS FOR CHILDREN

Oatmeal is known for its cardioprotective benefits From betaglucan fiber that lowers cholesterol, to the only antioxidants avantantamides that can help keep the walls of the vessels and lignans clean which are believed to protect against heart disease, are an attractive package. His basic porridge dish is practically a superhero.

BASIC OATS DURING THE NIGHT

+ ½ cup of gluten-free oatmeal or quinoa flakes
+ 1 tablespoon of ground flax seeds, chia seeds or hemp seeds
+ 1 tablespoon of maple syrup or coconut sugar (optional)
+ ¼ teaspoon ground cinnamon (optional)

FINISHING OPTIONS

+ 1 minced apple and 1 tablespoon of walnuts
+ 2 tablespoons of dried cranberries and 1 tablespoon of pumpkin seeds
+ 1 chopped pear and 1 spoonful of cashews
+ 1 cup of chopped grapes and 1 tablespoon of sunflower seeds
+
+ 1 sliced banana and 1 tablespoon of peanut butter
  2 tablespoons of raisins and 1 tablespoon of hazelnuts
+ 1 cup of blueberries and 1 tablespoon of sugarfree coconut flakes

1 Mix oatmeal, flax, maple syrup and cinnamon (if used) in a bowl or take them (travel mug or short thermos work very well)

2 Pour the oatmeal with enough cold water to dip it and mix to combine Soak for at least half an hour or overnight

3 Add the selection of your range

Quick option in the morning: boil about ½ cup of water and pour in the oatmeal Soak them for about 5 minutes before eating

Did you know that cinnamon has been shown **to** help control blood sugar, improve insulin response and reduce triglycerides, LDL cholesterol and bad total cholesterol?

Breakfast biscuits with oatmeal

Make 5 large cookies

Preparation time: 15 minutes / Cooking time: 12 minutes

QUICK PREPARATION FOR CHILDREN

Breakfast can be very healthy, even if you cook it in a biscuit Think of it as a healthy bowl of porridge, just more fun Oatmeal, flax seeds, walnuts and whole grains are beneficial for cardiovascular health, so these cookies are the perfect start to the day .Make them gluten free simply by using gluten free sorghum and oatmeal or quinoa flour instead of regular oatmeal.

- 1 **tablespoon of ground flax seeds**
- 2 **tablespoons of almond butter or sunflower butter**
- **2 tablespoons of maple syrup**
- **1 banana puree**
- **1 teaspoon ground cinnamon**
- **¼ teaspoon nutmeg powder (optional)**
- **A pinch of sea salt**
- **½ cup of oat flakes**
- **¼ cup raisins or dark chocolate chips**

1   Preheat the oven to 350 ° F Line a large baking tray with parchment paper

2   Mix the bedding with enough water to cover it with a saucer and set it aside

3   In a large bowl, mix the almond butter and maple syrup until a creamy consistency is obtained, then add the banana Add a mixture of flax and water

4   Change the cinnamon, nutmeg and salt to a separate medium bowl, then mix with a moist mixture 5 Add oatmeal and raisins and double

6 Form a ball with 3-4 tablespoons of pasta and press lightly to flatten the pan Repeat the operation, setting the cookies 2 to 3 inches apart

7 Cook for 12 minutes or until golden brown

8 Store the cookies in an airtight container in the refrigerator or freeze them for later

Go ahead: this amount is for one person, so you don't have many cookies to tempt yourself But they are excellent for doubling the entire batch of snacks

Sunshine Muffins

Make 6 cupcakes

Preparation time: 15 minutes / Cooking time: 30 minutes

FAST IMMEDIATE IMMEDIATE PREPARATION AMPLIFIER FOR CHILDREN

These cupcakes are the perfect start to the day, rich in flavor and nutrients. They have a very low content of added fats and sugars, based on the healthy sweetness of the fruit. If you want to be a little more sweet, add a few tablespoons of maple syrup with molasses .Try combining the muffin with half a cocktail to get a balanced breakfast.

- 1 teaspoon of coconut oil to distribute the muffin molds (optional)
- 2 tablespoons of almond butter or sunflower butter
- ¼ cup of raw milk
- 1 peeled orange
- 1carrot, cut into large pieces
- 2tablespoons chopped dried apricots or other dried fruit
- 3tbsp molasses
- 2 tablespoons of ground flax seeds
- 1 teaspoon apple cider vinegar
- 1 teaspoon pure vanilla extract
- ½ teaspoon of ground cinnamon
- ½ teaspoon ginger powder (optional)
- ¼ teaspoon nutmeg powder (optional)
- ¼ teaspoon of allspice (optional)
- ¾ cup of oatmeal or whole wheat flour
- 1 teaspoon of baking powder
- ½ teaspoon of baking soda

MIXTURES (OPTIONAL)

+ **½ cup of oat flakes**
+ **2 tablespoons of raisins or other chopped dried fruits**
+ **2 spoons of sunflower seeds**

1   Preheat the oven to 350 ° F Prepare a 6-cup muffin bowl by rubbing the inside of the cups with coconut oil or using silicone cups or paper cupcakes

2   In the food processor, clean peanut butter, milk, orange, carrots, apricots, molasses, flax seeds, vinegar, vanilla, cinnamon, ginger, nutmeg and allspice in the food processor or blender until smooth

3   Grind the oatmeal in a clean coffee grinder until it has the consistency of the flour (or use the whole wheat flour) In a large bowl, mix the oatmeal with the baking powder and baking soda

4   Mix the wet ingredients with the dry ingredients until combined Fold the accessories (if you use them)

5   Cook about ¼ cup of pasta on each roll and cook for 30 minutes or until the rod inserted inside is clean Orange creates a very moist base, so that the rolls can take longer than 30 minutes, depending on how heavy the muffin bowl is

<u>Inventories:</u> <u>keep the muffins in the refrigerator or freezer because they are very wet If you plan on keeping them frozen, you can easily double the batch of a full dozen</u>
Applesauce Crumble Muffins

Makes 12 cupcakes

Preparation time: 15 minutes / Cooking time: 15 to 20 minutes
QUICK PREPARATION FOR CHILDREN

They are adapted from my favorite sandwiches from my childhood to be completely vegetable and low in fat and sugar .Coconut sugar is an excellent choice for a low glycemic index sweetener, but if you can't find it, choose unprocessed brown sugar, such as sucanate, date sugar or other unrefined icing sugar .Do not use brown sugar, which is only refined white sugar with the addition of molasses Muskado, demerara or turbinado sugars are only partially refined, so it would be goo.d

- **1 teaspoon of coconut oil to distribute the muffin molds (optional)**
- **2 tablespoons of peanut butter or seed butter**
- **1½ cup unsweetened apple mousse**
- **⅓cup of coconut sugar**
- **½ cup of raw milk**
- **2 tablespoons of ground flax seeds**
- **1 teaspoon apple cider vinegar**
- **1 teaspoon pure vanilla extract**
- **2 cups of whole wheat flour**
- **1 teaspoon of baking soda**
- **½ teaspoon of baking powder**
- **1 teaspoon ground cinnamon**
- **A pinch of sea salt**
- **½ cup of chopped walnuts**
- **Ingredients (optional)**
- **¼ cup of walnuts**
- **¼ cup of coconut sugar**
- **½ teaspoon of ground cinnamon**

1 Preheat the oven to 350 ° F Prepare two 6-cup muffin trays by rubbing the inside of the cups with coconut oil or using silicone cups or paper cups

2In a large bowl, mix peanut butter, apple mousse, coconut sugar, milk, flaxseed, vinegar and vanilla until well mixed or cleaned in a robot for cooking or in a blender

3   In another large bowl, sift the flour, baking soda, baking powder, cinnamon, salt and chopped walnuts

4   Mix the dry ingredients with the wet ingredients until combined

5   Put about 1/4 cup of dough on each muffin and sprinkle with the coating of your choice (if using). Cook for 15-20 minutes or until the inner stick is clean. Apple compote creates a very moist base, so muffins can last longer, depending on the weight of the cans.

Options: To do this without nuts, replace the nuts with sunflower seeds and use sunflower seed butter

Baked French Banana Toast with Raspberry Syrup

Makes 8 slices

Preparation time: 10 minutes / Cooking time: 30 minutes

QUICK PREPARATION WITHOUT FRIENDS FRIENDS FOR CHILDREN

Preparing a French toast with bananas instead of eggs gives it a natural sweetness and a new flavor, and you don't have to worry about cooking it a little .The beauty of this raspberry syrup lies in the fact that the sweetness of the berries means that you only need a small amount of maple syrup, which reduces the amount of added sugar.

French toast

- 1 banana
- 1 cup of coconut milk
- 1 teaspoon pure vanilla extract
- ¼ teaspoon nutmeg powder
- ½ teaspoon of ground cinnamon
- 1½ teaspoon of arrowroot powder or flour
- A pinch of sea salt
- 8 slices of whole wheat bread

FOR RASPBERRY SYRUP

1 cup of fresh or frozen raspberries or other berries

2 tablespoons of water or pure fruit juice

1 or 2 tablespoons of maple syrup or coconut sugar (optional)

MAKING FRENCH TOASTED BREAD

1 Preheat the oven to 350 ° F.

2 In a shallow bowl, grate or grate the banana well Mix coconut milk, vanilla, nutmeg, cinnamon, carrots and salt.

3 Dip the slices of bread in the banana mixture, then put them in a 13 by 9-inch pan They should cover the bottom of the plate and may overlap slightly, but should not overlap. Pour the bread with the remaining banana and put the dish in the oven. Cook for about 30 minutes or until the top is slightly golden brown.

4 Serve with raspberry syrup.

TO MAKE RASPBERRY SYRUP

1   Heat the raspberries in a small saucepan with water and maple syrup (if used) over medium heat

2   Cook over low heat, stirring occasionally and breaking the berries, for 15-20 minutes until the liquid is reduced

<u>Leftovers:</u> <u>residual raspberry syrup is the perfect complement to simple oatmeal as a breakfast or a quick and delicious season with wholemeal toast with natural peanut butter</u>

Toast with apple and cinnamon

Make 2 slices

Preparation time: 5 minutes / Cooking time: 10 to 20 minutes

QUICK PREPARATION WITHOUT FRIENDS FRIENDS FOR CHILDREN

It is a very simple form of a decadent brunch Apples help regulate blood sugar levels, reduce fat and cholesterol and also help maintain the balance of intestinal flora .In apples there is a phytonutrient called quercetin, which has anti-inflammatory and antihistamine properties and is much more concentrated in the skin than in the flesh .In fact, there are several nutrients in apples that focus on the skin, so be sure to eat them.

- **1-2 teaspoons of coconut oil**
- **½ teaspoon of ground cinnamon**
- **1 tablespoon of maple syrup or coconut sugar**
- 1 **apple, heartless and finely chopped**

2 **slices of whole wheat bread**

1In a large bowl, mix coconut oil, cinnamon and maple syrup Add the apple slices and mix with your hands to cover them

2 To fry the toast, place the apple slices in a medium skillet over medium heat and cook for about 5 minutes until they are slightly soft, then transfer them to the plate. Bake the bread in the same pan for 2-3 minutes on each side Cover the toast with the apples Alternatively, you can prepare a toast Use your hand to rub each piece of bread with a small mixture of coconut oil on both sides. Place them on a baking sheet, cover with coated apples and put them in the oven or toaster at 350 ° F for 15-20 minutes or until the apples are tender.

Options: for a more daily version, bake the bread, spread with peanut butter, cover with apple slices and sprinkle a pinch of cinnamon and coconut sugar

Bowl of muesli and blueberries

Makes about 5 cups

Preparation time: 10 minutes

QUICK PREPARATION FOR CHILDREN

Muesli is an excellent alternative to muesli; It has less fat and does not cook In health food stores you will find whole and swollen flakes: look for the least amount of ingredients and without added sugar. It is a really tasty and energizing breakfast on weekdays as an alternative to oatmeal or cocktails. Have fun experimenting with various nuts, seeds, fruits and spices they may contain.

For SAMPLE

+ **1 cup of oatmeal**
+ **1 cup of spelled, quinoa or more oatmeal**
+ **2 cups of swollen cereals**

- ¼ cup of sunflower seeds
- ¼ cup of almonds
- ¼ cup of raisins
- ¼ cup of dried cranberries
- ¼ cup of chopped dried figs
- ¼ cup unsweetened grated coconut
- ¼ cup of non-dairy chocolate pieces
- 1-3 teaspoons of ground cinnamon

FOR CUENCO

- ½ cup of unsweetened milk or apple mousse
- ¾ cup of muesli
- ½ cup of berries

1 Place the muesli ingredients in the bowl or bag and shake.

2 Combine the muesli ingredients and the bowl in a bowl or on a takeaway plate.

<u>**Substitutions:**</u> <u>try Brazil nuts, peanuts, dried cranberries, dried cranberries, dried mangoes or whatever inspires you Ginger and cardamom are interesting flavors if you want to branch with spices</u>

Quinoa and chocolate breakfast bowl

Make 2 portions

Preparation time: 5 minutes / Cooking time: 30 minutes
QUICK PREPARATION GLUTEN FREE WITHOUT CHILDREN FRIENDS

At breakfast you can enjoy completely healthy desserts Quinoa is excellent for adding a morning protein enhancer, but you can use any cooked whole wheat, from oatmeal to brown rice .The pudding is also excellent as a snack or dessert for making chocolate.

- **1 cup of quinoa**
- **1 teaspoon ground cinnamon**
- **1 cup of milk without milk**
- **1 cup of water**
- **1 large banana**
- **2-3 tablespoons of bitter or carob cocoa powder**
- **1 or 2 tablespoons of almond butter or other peanut butter or seed butter**
- **1 tablespoon of ground flax seeds or chia or hemp seeds**
- **2 spoons of walnuts**
- **¼ cup of raspberries**

1   Put quinoa, cinnamon, milk and water in a medium saucepan Bring to a boil over high heat, then lower the temperature and simmer for 25-30 minutes

2   While cooking the quinoa, mix or grate the banana in a medium bowl and add cocoa powder, almond butter and flax seeds

3   To serve, pour 1 cup of cooked quinoa into a bowl, cover with half pudding, half walnuts and raspberries

Prepare in advance: This is a great way to use leftovers from quinoa or plan ahead and prepare additional quinoa for dinner, so you can prepare it in the morning from Monday to Friday, as soon as with a smoothie

Carrot and ginger soup

It produces 3 to 4 large bowls

Preparation time: 10 minutes / Cooking time: 20 minutes

QUICK PREPARATION GLUTEN FREE

Carrot and ginger soup is quick and easy to prepare during the week, it is also nutritious and really tasty. Carrots are always associated with good vision due to the high beta-carotene content, but carrots have also been shown to have antioxidants and other nutrients to protect against cardiovascular disease, cancer and liver problems .The addition of white beans (I mentioned cannellini beans here, which are white beans, but will work with any type of white beans) makes the soup full, thick, creamy and rich in protein.

+ **1 teaspoon of olive oil**
+ **1 cup chopped onion**
+ **1 tablespoon chopped fresh ginger**
+ **4 large carrots, peeled or rubbed and chopped (about 2 cups)**
+ **1 cup of boiled or canned cannellini beans and rinsed or other soft white beans**
+ **½ cup of vegetable broth or water and additional salt**
+ **2 glasses of water**
+ **¼ teaspoon of sea salt**

1   Heat the olive oil in a large saucepan, then fry the onion and ginger for 2-3 minutes .Add the carrots and cook until tender, about 3 minutes.

2   Add beans, vegetable broth, water and salt and simmer for 20 minutes.

3   Transfer the soup to a blender or use an immersion blender to crush Serve hot.

Leftovers: store the **leftovers** in an airtight container in the refrigerator for a week or in the freezer for one to two months

Coconut soup with watercress

Makes 4 bowls

Preparation time: 10 minutes / Cooking time: 20 minutes

QUICK REINFORCEMENT WITHOUT RAPID IMPULSING PREPARATION THE IMMUNITY ANTI-FLAMMATORY

Such mixed soups are the perfect way to collect many incognito vegetables. This soup is so delicious that no one complains about eating vegetables and its creaminess is sweet and the alcohol of coconut milk compensates for the bitterness of watercress .To make this recipe raw, use 2-3 dishes instead of frying regular onions and stir the soup when it is cold.

- **1 teaspoon of coconut oil**
- **1 chopped onion**
- **2 cups of fresh or frozen peas**
- **4 cups of water or vegetable broth**
- **1 cup fresh cress, chopped**
- **1 tablespoon chopped fresh mint**
- **A pinch of sea salt**
- **A pinch of freshly ground black pepper**
  ¾ cup of coconut milk

1   Dissolve the coconut oil in a large saucepan over medium heat .Add the onions and cook until tender, about 5 minutes, then add the peas and water.

2   Bring to a boil, then lower the heat and add watercress, mint, salt and pepper Cover and simmer for 5 minutes.

3   Add the coconut milk and mix the soup until smooth in a blender or hand blender.

Beetroot and sweet potato soup

6 bowls ago

Preparation time: 10 minutes / Cooking time: 30 minutes

FAST PREPARATION GLUTEN FREE pleasant for children Anti-inflammatory immunity enhancer

This potato and beetroot soup recipe is easy to prepare and has an extraordinary flavor .The combination of beetroot and sweet potato offers a rich flavor and a thick, creamy consistency .The soup has a nice beetroot color and is very hot on a cold afternoon.

- **5 cups of unsalted water or vegetable broth (if salty, skip the sea salt below)**
- **1-2 teaspoons of olive oil or vegetable broth**
- **1 cup chopped onion**
- **3 minced garlic cloves**
- **1 tablespoon thyme, fresh or dried**
- **1-2 teaspoons of pepper**
- **2 cups of peeled and chopped beets**
- **2 cups of peeled and chopped sweet potatoes**
- **2 cups of peeled and chopped parsnips**
- **½ teaspoon of sea salt**
- **1 cup of chopped fresh mint**
- **½ avocado or 2 tablespoons of peanut butter or seed butter (optional)**
- **2 tablespoons of balsamic vinegar (optional)**
- **2 tablespoons of pumpkin seeds**

1 Boil the water in a large pot.

2

Heat another olive oil in a large pot and fry the onion and garlic until tender, about 5 minutes.

3 Add thyme, peppers, beets, sweet potatoes and parsnips, along with boiling water and salt .Cover and simmer for about 30 minutes until the vegetables are soft.

4 Reserve a little mint for decoration and add the rest along with the avocado (if in use) Stir until well mixed.

5 Transfer the soup to a blender or use a puree immersion blender, adding balsamic vinegar (if used).

6 Serve with pumpkin seeds and fresh mint, and perhaps with pieces of the other half of avocado, if used.

Leftovers: this soup is ideal for preparing large quantities and storing in single-dose containers in the freezer for quick meals during the week

Miso Soup with Noodles

Makes 4 bowls

Preparation time: 10 minutes / Cooking time: 15 minutes

GLUTEN-FREE PREPARATION WITH ANTIINFLAMMATORY WALNUT

Miso soup is Japanese and is traditionally served in the simplest way possible: broth, miso, hijiki seaweed, tofu cubes and shallots Many Japanese miso soups will also contain sardines and tuna in broth, but we will keep them herbal .We also take a fusion approach, combining the concept of North American chicken noodle soup with Japanese ingredients, using azuki beans and earthy soba noodles to clean (Soba usually comes in small packages in one package and 7 ounces are approximately two packages in a typical package).

- **7 ounces of soba paste (use 100% gluten-free buckwheat)**
- **4 glasses of water**
- **4 spoons of miso**
- **1 cup of azuki beans (boiled or canned), drained and rinsed**
- **2 tablespoons of fresh coriander or finely chopped basil**
- **2 shallots, finely chopped**

1 Boil a large pot of water, then add the Soba noodles Stir occasionally; Cooking will take about 5 minutes.

In the meantime, prepare the rest of the soup by heating the water in a separate pan just below the boil, then remove from the heat Stir the miso in water until it dissolves.

3 After cooking the pasta, filter and rinse with hot water.

4 Add the boiled noodles, azuki beans, coriander and chives to the miso broth and serve.

Technique: Miso is a fermented product and good brands have live microbial cultures, such as

yogurt, so it should be added to the broth when it is hot, not hot Adding miso to boiling water changes the flavor

Creamy pumpkin soup with toasted walnuts

Makes 4 bowls

Preparation time: 15 minutes / Cooking time: 30 minutes

RAPID REINFORCEMENT WITHOUT GLUTEN WITHOUT ANTI-INFLAMMATORY PREPARATION OF THE IMMUNE BOOSTER

It is the perfect soup to warm and satisfy it, helping the body to purify itself. It is very tasty and very rich, but it makes those concentrations of books feel .It is a perfect spirit book for spiritual meals after the holidays, when we ate and desired too much the day before.

+ **1 small pumpkin pie, peeled, sown and chopped (about 6 cups)**
+ **1 teaspoon of olive oil**
+ **¼ teaspoon of sea salt**
+ **1 chopped onion**
+ **4 cups of water or vegetable broth**
+ **2-3 teaspoons of ground sage**
+ **2-3 tablespoons of yeast**
+ **1 cup of milk or 1 tablespoon of peanut butter or seed butter plus 1 cup of water or broth + ¼ cup of toasted walnuts**

Freshly ground black pepper

1) Put a large saucepan over medium heat and fry the pumpkin in oil, season with salt until lightly tender, about 10 minutes .Add the onion to the pan and fry until tender, about 5 minutes.

Add water and boil. Then lower the temperature over low heat, cover and cook for 15-20 minutes until the pumpkin softens after the bite with a fork

3 Add sage, nourishing yeast and non-dairy milk .Then grate the soup with an immersion blender or in a normal blender until smooth

4 Garnish with roasted nuts and pepper.

Replacement: winter squash or sweet potato would be an excellent alternative to squash in terms of texture, flavor and nutrients

Roasted pepper and pumpkin soup

6 bowls ago

Preparation time: 10 minutes / Cooking time: 40 to 50 minutes

FAST PREPARATION GLUTEN FREE pleasant for children Anti-inflammatory immunity enhancer

Roasted vegetables attract sugars and give this soup its full flavor .The beauty of cooking vegetables is that although cooking takes time, you put them in the oven and you can do other things. It's great to have such a thick, creamy and tasty non-dairy soup.

- **1 small pumpkin**
- **1 tablespoon of olive oil**
- **1 teaspoon of sea salt**
- **2 red peppers**
- **1 yellow onion**
- **1 head of garlic**
- **2 cups of water or vegetable broth**
- **1 zest and lime juice**
- **1-2 tablespoons of Tahini**
- **A pinch of cayenne pepper**
- **½ teaspoon of coriander powder**
- **½ teaspoon ground cumin Roasted pumpkin seeds (optional)**

1 Preheat the oven to 350 ° F.

2 Prepare the roasted pumpkin, cutting it in half lengthwise, removing the seeds and making several holes in the meat with

a fork Book the seeds if you wish .Rub a small amount of oil on the meat and skin, then rub with a little sea salt and place the halves with the skin facing downwards in a large pan .Put in the oven, preparing the rest of the vegetables.

3 Prepare the peppers in exactly the same way, except that it is not necessary to cut them .Cut the onion in half and rub the oil on the exposed faces. Cut the tip of the garlic and rub the oil on the exposed meat.

4 After cooking the pumpkin for 20 minutes, add the paprika, onion and garlic and cook for another 20 minutes. Optionally, you can toast pumpkin seeds by placing them in the oven on a separate plateA dish 10 to 15 minutes before the vegetables are finished Look at them carefully.

5 After cooking the vegetables, remove them and let them cool before handling them .The pumpkin will be very soft after the piercing with a fork.

6 Remove the meat from the pumpkin peel in a large saucepan (if you have an immersion blender) or in a blender. Chop the pepper roughly, remove the onion peel and chop the onion approximately and squeeze the garlic cloves from the head, all in a pot or blender Add water, lemon zest and juice and tahini .Grate the soup, if necessary, add more water to the desired consistency.

7 Season with salt, pepper, coriander and cumin Serve garnished with roasted pumpkin seeds (if used).

<u>Did you know that</u> <u>winter squash has a lot of vitamin A, which is good for eye health and skin repair and maintenance? It also stimulates the immune system According to Chinese medicine, winter squash improves the circulation of qi energy, which is its life force</u>

Weekday tomato and chickpea soup

Make 2 portions

Preparation time: 10 minutes / Cooking time: 20 minutes

NOTE GLUTEN FREE WITHOUT IMMUNITY RAPID WHEAT PREPARATIONS

This soup is quick and easy to prepare, as well as super tasty, with some rich and wonderful flavors. It is perfect for a quick dinner during the week and enough for lunch the next day .If you cook for two or more, the recipe will easily double or triple.

- **1-2 teaspoons of olive oil or vegetable broth**
- **½ cup of chopped onion**
- **3 minced garlic cloves**
- **1 cup of chopped mushrooms**
- **⅛ to ¼ teaspoon of sea salt, divided**
- **1 tablespoon of dried basil**
- **½ tablespoon of dried oregano**
- **1 or 2 tablespoons of balsamic vinegar or red wine**
  1 can of diced tomatoes
- **1 can (14 ounces) of chickpeas, drained and rinsed or 1 cup of cooked lubricant**
- **2 glasses of water**
- **1 or 2 cups of chopped cabbage**
1 Heat a large olive oil in a large saucepan and fry the onion, garlic and mushrooms with a pinch of salt until tender, for 7 to 8 minutes.

2 Add basil and oregano and stir to mix .Then add the vinegar to defrost the pan with a wooden spoon to scrape all the salty and golden pieces from the bottom.

3   Add tomatoes and chickpeas .Mix, combine, add enough water to obtain the desired consistency.

4   Add the cabbage and the remaining salt .Cover and simmer for 5-15 minutes until the cabbage is as soft as you want.

<u>Salsa: it</u> <u>is delicious covered with a spoonful of toasted walnuts and a pinch of nutritious yeast</u> <u>or sprinkled cheese</u>

Abundant chili

Makes 4 bowls

Preparation time: 10 minutes / Cooking time: 10 to 20 minutes

RAPID   REINFORCEMENT   RAPID IMMUNE REINFORCEMENT

Beans are an excellent source of protein, which contain fiber, folic acid, iron and manganese, which lower cholesterol and stabilize blood sugar, without saturated fat and ground beef cholesterol .The combination of iron-rich beans with tomatoes rich in vitamin C and coriander means that .Poch is more desired than iron, which correlates with greater energy.

- **1 chopped onion**
- **2-3 cloves of minced garlic**
- **1 teaspoon of olive oil or 1 or 2 tablespoons of water, vegetable broth or red wine**
- **1 can of tomatoes (28 ounces)**
- **¼ cup of tomato paste or crushed tomatoes**

+ **1 can (14 ounces) of beans, rinsed and dried or 1 ½ cup of cooking**
+ **2-3 teaspoons of chili powder**
+ **¼ teaspoon of sea salt**
+ **¼ cup of fresh coriander leaves or parsley leaves**

1 Fry the onion and garlic in oil in a large saucepan for about 5 minutes .After softening, add the tomatoes, tomato paste, beans and chilli powder Season with salt.

2 Boil on low heat for at least 10 minutes or for as long as you wish .The flavors will improve, the longer they cook over low heat and even better, like leftovers. 3 Decorate with coriander and serve.

Options: Other beans have similar nutrients, so you can change them if you wish Try black beans, adzuki or dark beans Season with spicy sauce if necessary

Indian red lentil soup

Makes 4 bowls

Preparation time: 5 minutes / Cooking time: 50 minutes

QUICK REINFORCEMENT WITHOUT RAPID IMPULSING PREPARATION THE IMMUNITY ANTIFLAMMATORY

It is a rich and abundant soup with a bold and warm taste of fresh ginger, as well as Indian spices such as coriander, cumin and turmeric .Sweet potatoes are rich in vitamin A, add a delicate sweetness to counter the spices and, as a vegetable root, help to grind and concentrate the mind.

- 1 cup of red lentils
- 2 glasses of water
- 1 teaspoon curry powder plus 1 tbsp, split or 5 coriander seeds (optional)
- 1 teaspoon of coconut oil or 1 tablespoon of water or vegetable broth
- 1 red onion, diced
- 1 tablespoon chopped fresh ginger
- 2 cups of sweet potatoes, peeled and diced
- 1 cup of sliced zucchini
- Freshly ground black pepper
- Sea salt
- 3-4 glasses of vegetable broth or water
- 1 or 2 teaspoons of toasted sesame oil
- 1 bunch of chopped spinach
  Toast with sesame

1 Put the lentils in a large pot with 2 glasses of water and 1 teaspoon of curry powder .Bring the lentils to a boil, then reduce the heat and simmer for 10 minutes until the lentils are soft.

2 In the meantime, heat a large saucepan over medium heat Add the coconut oil and fry the onions and ginger until tender, about 5 minutes. Add the sweet potato and leave it on the fire for about 10 minutes to soften it a bit, then add the courgettes and cook until it appears bright, about 5 minutes. Add the remaining 1 tablespoon of curry powder, pepper and salt and mix the vegetables to cover.

3 Add the vegetable stock, boil, then simmer and cover Cook the vegetables slowly for 20-30 minutes or until the sweet potato softens.

4 Add the cooked lentils to the soup Add another pinch of salt, roasted sesame oil and spinach Stir, allowing the spinach to dry before removing the pan from the heat.

5 Serve with toasted sesame seeds.

Did you know that orange pulp sweet potatoes are the tastiest and are often called sweet potatoes, even though the white and orange varieties are technically sweet potatoes? True yams are tropical tubers and are generally not sold in North America

Lentil curry burger

It produces 12 hamburgers

Preparation time: 40 minutes / Cooking time: 30 to 40 minutes

Anti-inflammatory immunity enhancer GLUTEN FREE

When I started making veggie burgers, I tried to get a good consistency that was good to sustain, but not too heavy I tried many recipes before combining some aspects in my version, using carrots and many spices to lighten lentils .These burgers are dense and abundant, with tons of flavor and nutritional value.

- **1 cup of lentils**
- **2½ to 3 glasses of water**
- **3 grated carrots**
- **1 small onion, diced**

- ¾ cup of whole wheat flour (see gluten-free options below)
- 1½ or 2 teaspoons of curry powder
- ½ teaspoon of sea salt
- A pinch of freshly ground black pepper

1   Put the lentils in a medium bowl with water Bring to a boil and then simmers for about 30 minutes until smooth.

2   While cooking the lentils, put the carrots and onions in a large bowl Mix with flour, curry, salt and pepper.

3   When the lentils are cooked, drain the excess water, then add them to the bowl with the vegetables .Use a meat grinder or large spoon to gently mash them and add more flour if you want the mixture to stick .The amount of flour depends on the amount of water absorbed by the lentils and the consistency of the flour, so use it approximately until the mixture adheres when the ball is formed Eliminate 1/4 of service and create 12 empanadas.

4You can fry or cook hamburgers .To fry, heat a large pan over medium heat, add a little oil and cook the hamburgers for about 10 minutes on the first page. Turn and cook another 5-7 minutes To cook them, put them on a baking sheet lined with parchment and cook at 350 ° F for 30 to 40 minutes.

Options: for wholemeal flour, use the desired flour Sorghum, rice, oats, buckwheat and even

<u>almond flour would work to make them gluten-</u>

<u>free The flour of this recipe is only a folder, so it</u>

<u>can be of any type</u>
Dijon Maple Burger

It produces 12 hamburgers

Preparation time: 20 minutes / Cooking time: 30 minutes

REFLECTIVE AMPLIFIER FOR CHILDREN

A lot of fun in vegetarian burgers comes from what you decide to spend. You can mix and match the hamburger with the dressing, based on the flavors of the hamburger .They go well with pieces of marinade, avocado, cherry tomatoes and lettuce.

- **1 red pepper**
- **1 can of chickpeas, rinsed and dried or 2 cooked cups**
- **1 cup of chopped almonds**
- **2 teaspoons of Dijon mustard**
- **2 teaspoons of maple syrup**
- **1 clove of garlic, pressed**
- **½ lemon juice**
- **1 teaspoon dried oregano**
- **½ teaspoon dry sage**
- **1 cup of spinach**
- **1 to 1½ cup of oat flakes**

1   Preheat the oven to 350 ° F .Line a large baking tray with parchment paper.

2   Cut the pepper in half, remove the stem and seeds, then place the pan with the cut side facing up in the oven. Cook, preparing the remaining ingredients.

3   Put the chickpeas in the food processor together with almonds, mustard, maple syrup, garlic, lemon juice, oregano, sage and spinach .Press until everything comes together but it's clean .When the pepper softens a little, about 10 minutes, add it to the processor along with the oatmeal flakes and press until they are cut enough to create empanadas.

4   If you don't have a food processor, mash the chickpeas with a meat grinder or fork and make sure that everything else is chopped as finely as possible, then mix.

5   Cut 1/4 cup portions and form 12 empanadas and place them on a baking sheet.

6   Put the hamburgers in the oven and cook until lightly browned, for about 30 minutes.

__Technique: It is important__ not to rub the ingredients because you want a consistency for your burgers, not porridge Use short pulses in the processor until the ingredients are minced

Burger Cajun

It produces from 5 to 6 hamburgers

Preparation time: 25 minutes / Cooking time: 10 to 30 minutes

GLUTEN FREE ANTI-FLAMMABLE WITHOUT NUT

These burgers are made with toasted buckwheat (also known as porridge), which has a flavonoid called rutin, contains vegetable lignans and is a good source of magnesium, all cardio protective Buckwheat nutrients can also help control blood sugar levels .Combine this nutrition with incredible flavors, turn it into a hamburger and you will have one of the best meals.

DRESSED
- 1 tablespoon of Tahini
- 1 tablespoon of apple cider vinegar
- 2 teaspoons of Dijon mustard
- 1 or 2 spoons of water
- 1 or 2 pressed garlic cloves
- 1 teaspoon dried basil
- 1 teaspoon dried thyme
- ½ teaspoon dried oregano
- ½ teaspoon dry sage
- ½ teaspoon smoked paprika
- ¼ teaspoon cayenne pepper
- ¼ teaspoon of sea salt
- A pinch of freshly ground black pepper
- FOR HAMBURG
- 2 glasses of water
- 1 cup of semolina (toasted buckwheat)
- A pinch of sea salt
- 2 grated carrots
- A handful of chopped fresh parsley

1 teaspoon of olive oil (optional)   TO MAKE A COSTUME

1 In a medium bowl, mix tahin, vinegar and mustard until the mixture is very thick. Add 1 or 2 tablespoons of dilution water and beat again until smooth.

2 Add the rest of the ingredients Set aside the flavors to mix.

MAKE HAMBURG

1   Put water, buckwheat and sea salt in a medium saucepan Bring to a boil and simmer for 2-3 minutes, then simmer, cover and simmer for 15 minutes .Buckwheat is fully cooked when it is soft and there is no liquid on the bottom of the pan Do not mix buckwheat during cooking.

2   After cooking the buckwheat, transfer it to a large bowl .Mix grated carrots, fresh parsley and whole buckwheat sauce. Take ¼ cup to serve and shape the burgers.

3   You can fry or cook hamburgers .To fry, heat a large pan over medium heat, add 1 teaspoon of olive oil and cook the hamburgers for about 5 minutes on the first page .Turn and cook another 5 minutes .To cook them, place them on a baking sheet lined with parchment and cook at about 350 ° F for about 30 minutes.

You know that buckwheat isn't associated with wheat In fact, it is a grain and does not contain gluten .It also has a different nutritional profile than whole grains. Buckwheat is rich in lysine amino acids, which helps balance the diet of plants, because many plant foods are rich in other amino acids, but low in lysine Other lysinerich foods are beans and legumes, quinoa and pistachios

Grilled AHLT

Makes 1 sandwich

Preparation time: 5 minutes / Cooking time: 10 minutes

QUICK PREPARATION WITHOUT A FLAMMABLE SEARCH FOR CHILDREN

Give BLT a healthy and delicious touch by replacing the bacon with avocado and hummus .When I was grilled, I also swapped spinach for lettuce .You can also use the massaged cabbage if necessary, massaging it with your fingers until it dries and moistens a little .It is the perfect place for a quick dinner with some french fries.

- **¼ cup of classic hummus**
- **2 slices of whole wheat bread**
- **¼ of sliced avocado**
- **½ cup of chopped lettuce**
- **½ chopped tomato**
- **A pinch of sea salt**
- **A pinch of freshly ground black pepper**
- **1 teaspoon of olive oil, divided**

1   Spread a little humus on each slice of bread .Then put avocado, lettuce and tomato on a slice, sprinkle with salt and pepper and cover with the second slice.

2   Heat the pan over medium heat and sprinkle the asp with a teaspoon of olive oil just before putting the sandwich in the pan.

Cook for 3- 5 minutes, then lift the sandwich with a spatula, sprinkle the remaining half teaspoon of olive oil in a pan and turn the sandwich to cook on the other side for 3-5 minutes Press with a spatula to seal the vegetables inside.

3   When finished, remove it from the pan and cut it in half to serve.

Technique: you can also toast the bread and fold it like a simple sandwich or roll out the bread with olive oil, fold the sandwich and put it in a toaster for 10-15 minutes at 350 ° F

Black bean pizza loaded

Make 2 small pizzas

Preparation time: 10 minutes / Cooking time: 10 to 20 minutes

QUICK REINFORCEMENT WITHOUT FRIEND IMMUNITY FRIEND GLUTEN FREE

This pizza is not only super tasty, but also full of delicious fresh vegetables. You can cook it or try it with raw ingredients to give it a summer touch. Using bean sauce as a pizza sauce gives you a protein injection. You have many options for barking here Go to the shop with two hazelnuts or a complete package or create it yourself with the Easy DIY pizza dough or the Herbed Millet pizza dough, divided into two pizzas.

- **2 pizza bases ready**
- **½ cup spicy black bean sauce**
- **1 tomato, thinly sliced**
- **A pinch of freshly ground black pepper**
- **1 grated carrot**
- **A pinch of sea salt**
- **1 red onion, finely chopped**
- **1 sliced avocado**

1 Preheat the oven to 400 ° F

2 Place two skins on a large baking sheet Spread half the spicy black bean sauce on each pizza dough. Then, add the tomato layers with a pinch of pepper, if desired.

3 Sprinkle the grated carrot with sea salt and massage gently with your hands .Spread the carrot over the tomato, then add the onion.

4 Put the pizzas in the oven for 10-20 minutes or until they fit.

5 Cover the cooked pizza with sliced avocado and another pinch of pepper.

<u>Options:</u> <u>try making a fresh pizza without cooking Just load the pita or cook the skin before loading it and you can use asparagus instead of red Bonus points and flavor if they are covered with fresh alfalfa sprouts</u>

Mediterranean Hummus Pizza

Make 2 small pizzas

Preparation time: 10 minutes / Cooking time: 20 to 30 minutes

FAST PREPARATION GLUTEN FREE pleasant for children Anti-inflammatory immunity enhancer

This is one of his favorite meals for a week at home, because everything is available to the public and quickly prepared for a satisfying meal .Organize these pizzas above with vegetables: create the top you want, as much as you want .The olives give the pizza a tasty and tasty flavor, but if you don't want to try the chopped and sun-dried tomatoes. You can use two pizzas or a package of wholemeal crust or do it yourself with the Easy DIY pizza crust or the Herbed Millet pizza crust, divided into two pizzas.

+ **½ courgettes, finely chopped**
+ **½ red onion, finely chopped**
+ **1 cup of cherry tomatoes, cut in half**
+ **2-4 tablespoons of chopped and chopped black olives**
+ **A pinch of sea salt**
+ **Olive oil spray (optional)**
+ **2 pizza bases ready**
+ **½ cup of classic hummus or hummus of roasted red peppers**
+ **2-4 tablespoons of sprinkled cheese**

1 Preheat the oven to 400 ° F.

2 Put zucchini, onion, cherry tomatoes and olives in a large bowl, sprinkle with sea salt and mix lightly. Sprinkle some olive oil (if used) to preserve the flavor and prevent it from drying out in the oven.

3Place two skins on a large baking sheet .Spread half the humus on each skin and cover with a mixture of vegetables and a pinch of cheese flakes.

4 Put the pizza in the oven for 20-30 minutes or until the vegetables are soft.

Advancement: in short, gently fry the vegetables before putting them on the pizza, then you just have to cook them for a few minutes until they heat up .I could even use the remaining fried vegetables

Pack of chickpeas with curry mango

3 turns ago

Preparation time: 15 minutes

QUICK PREPARATION WITHOUT A FLAMMABLE SEARCH FOR CHILDREN

Sweet mango combined with curry and flavored with calciumrich tahini is perfection .Eat it for dinner; You can heat vegetables and chickpeas before putting them in the package, then packing leftovers for lunch during the trip. Just remember to bring your napkins because they are a little messy.

- 3 spoons of Tahini
- 1 zest and lime juice
- 1 tablespoon curry powder
- ¼ teaspoon of sea salt
- 3-4 tablespoons of water
- 1 can (14 ounces) of chickpeas, rinsed and dried, or 1 ½ cup of cooking
- 1 cup diced mango
- 1 red pepper, inoculated and diced
- ½ cup fresh coriander, chopped
- 3 large whole tablets

1-2 cups of grated green lettuce

1   In a medium bowl, mix tahin, zest and lime juice, curry and salt until the mixture is creamy and thick Add 3-4 tablespoons of water to dilute it a little .Or you can process everything in a blender. The taste should be strong and salty to flavor the whole salad.

2   Mix the chickpeas, mango, pepper and coriander with the tahini sauce.

3	Cover the salad in the center of the package, cover with the chopped lettuce, then roll up and taste.

Options: replace lettuce leaves with integrated wrappers Use a hard lettuce, such as Boston, Bibb or butter lettuce, or place the filling on the escarole leaves if it matches the slightly bitter taste

Falafel package

It produces 6 cakes, 1 pack

Preparation time: 30 minutes / Cooking time: 30 to 40 minutes

NO NUTS an immune system stimulator suitable for children

Falafel and hummus are probably the two most popular chickpea dishes in global cuisine, so combine them. Fill the falafel with nutrient-rich additives, such as parsley and cook or fry, instead of frying for vegetable benefits. This recipe is for wrapping, but since falafel takes time, the recipe has six cakes, enough for six wraps .Just do more wraps for the whole band, or I'll give you some advice on what to do with the remaining falafel.

FOR FALAFEL POTATOES
- **1 can (14 ounces) of chickpeas, drained and rinsed or 1 cup of cooked lubricant**
- **1 grated zucchini**
- **2 chopped chives**
- **¼ cup of fresh parsley, chopped**
- **2 tablespoons of black olives, pitted and chopped (optional)**
- **1 tablespoon of tahini or almond butter, cashews or sunflower seeds**
- **1 tablespoon of lemon juice or apple cider vinegar**
- **½ teaspoon ground cumin**
- **¼ teaspoon pepper**
- **¼ teaspoon of sea salt**
- **1 teaspoon of olive oil (optional, if fried)**

To wrap

- 1 integrated package or pita
- ¼ cup of classic hummus
- ½ cup of fresh vegetables
- 1 baked falafel cake
- ¼ cup of cherry tomatoes cut in half
- ¼ cup diced cucumber
- ¼ cup chopped avocado or guacamole
- ¼ cup quinoa salad or cooked taboule (optional)

MAKE A FAILURE

1Use a food processor to increase chickpeas, courgettes, shallots, parsley and olives (if used) until cut. Just press, don't delete. Or use a meat grinder to mix chickpeas in a large bowl and add grated and chopped vegetables.

2	In a small bowl, mix the tahin and lemon juice and add cumin, pepper and salt Pour it into the chickpea mixture and mix well (or press the food processor) to combine. Try adding more salt if you need it Use your hands to form a mixture in 6 empanadas.

3	You can fry or cook the cake .To fry, heat a large pan over medium heat, add 1 teaspoon of olive oil and cook the cake for about 10 minutes on the first page. Turn and cook another 5-7 minutes To cook them, put them on a baking sheet lined with parchment and cook at 350 ° F for 30 to 40 minutes.

To wrap

1	Place the package on a plate and distribute the hummus in the center. Then lie down on the green and crumble the falafel cake on top .Add tomatoes, cucumbers, avocados and quinoa.

2   Fold both ends and wrap them as tightly as possible If you have a sandwich press, you can press the pack for about 5 minutes It will be best to travel in a reusable container or reusable plastic packaging.

Inventories: Store the remaining empanadas in a sealed container in the refrigerator for a week or in the freezer for up to two months Take them as a hamburger, season with your favorite spices (vegetables and beans combine very well), mash them with lettuce or as separate cakes with a creamy avocado salad

Pad Thai Bowl

Makes 2 bowls

Preparation time: 10 minutes / Cooking time: 10 minutes

GLUTEN Quick Prep Immune Booster

Thai rootstock is usually prepared with eggs and fish sauce, making it difficult for plant eaters to find a solution. However, don't worry, because you can create your own and saturate so much flavor that you prefer compared to the restaurant version. In addition, you can pack many fresh and tasty vegetables to increase nutrient density Instead of the usual peanuts on top, you can pour this kind of peanuts directly into the sauce and drink it.

- **7 ounces of brown rice noodles**
- **1 teaspoon of olive oil or 1 tablespoon of vegetable broth or water**
- **2 carrots, peeled or rubbed and chopped in julienne**
- **1 cup finely chopped napa or red cabbage**
- **1 red pepper, sown and finely chopped**
- **2 shallots, finely chopped**
- **2-3 tablespoons of fresh mint, finely chopped**
- **1 cup of bean sprouts**
- **¼ cup of peanut sauce**
- **¼ cup chopped fresh coriander**
- **2 tablespoons of toasted peanuts, chopped Fresh lime wedges**

1 Place the rice noodles in a large bowl or saucepan and cover with boiling water. Leave to soften for about 10 minutes Rinse, filter and cool.

Heat the oil in a medium-high pan and fry the carrots, cabbage and pepper until tender, 7 to 8 minutes .Add the shallot, mint and bean sprouts and cook for a minute or two, then remove from the heat.

3 Mix the pasta with the vegetables and mix with a nut sauce.

4 Transfer to bowls and sprinkle with coriander and peanuts.

 Serve with a slice of lime to squeeze on a plate to give it a gustatory note.

Options: to try an even richer version of this bowl, skip the rice noodles and peel them or turn the zucchini or carrot into long "spaghetti"

A bowl of miso-coconut dragon

1 bowl ago

Preparation time: 10 minutes / Cooking time: 20 minutes

RAPID PREPARATION WITHOUT ANTIINFLAMMATORY GLUTEN INCREASE

This salty and creamy bowl is easy to prepare, but tasty and nutritious It does not contain oil, but the fat content of coconut milk makes months satisfactory .The selection of varieties of coconut milk with a low COG of spirit of fats names in the order of right, COG is looking for the cans of the yellow corners containing only coconut water and rubber. Composition of ingredients of chewing gum Guar gum is a soluble fiber derived from plants that helps to thicken the coconut milk filters when part of the fat.

FOR CUENCO
+ 1 **teaspoon of coconut oil or vegetable broth or water**
+ **½ red onion, finely chopped**
+ **A pinch of sea salt**
+ **½ cup of chopped brown mushrooms**
½ cup of cherry tomatoes, cut in half

DRESSED
+ 2 **spoons of fresh mint, finely chopped**
+ **¼ cup of canned coconut milk**
+ **1-2 teaspoons of miso paste**
+ **1 teaspoon of coconut sugar or maple syrup (optional)**

TO SERVE

+ **¾ cup of cooked quinoa, millet, brown rice or other whole grains**
+ **1 cup rocket or spinach (if ripe, chopped leaves)**
+ **1 tablespoon of chopped almonds**

1   Heat the oil in a medium skillet over medium heat and lightly fry the onion with salt for about 5 minutes .Add the mushrooms and cook until they are completely soft .Then add the cherry tomatoes and cook until tender, about 10 minutes in total.

2   Prepare the sauce by mixing or mixing the mint, coconut milk, miso paste and coconut sugar or maple syrup (if used) in a medium bowl. Add this to the cooked vegetables and then remove from the heat.

3   Serve the boiled vegetables on top of the quinoa, with the rocket on top and the almonds to decorate.

<u>Options: you can use green or red curry paste instead of miso in a delicious curry bowl</u>

A bowl of Soba noodles with cashews and ginger

Makes 2 bowls

Preparation time: 5 minutes / Cooking time: 20 minutes

GLUTEN Quick Prep Immune Booster

It is a delicious dish that is served cold in summer or warm in winter Soba is a thin Japanese buckwheat noodle, so it usually doesn't contain gluten .But check the ingredients, because some soba noodles can also use wheat flour .If you can't find or like soba noodles, try udon noodles or brown rice .In Japan, drinking these pastas is socially acceptable, especially if you eat hot Hide, people.

In the balls

- 7 ounces of soba paste
- 1 carrot, peeled or rubbed and cut into julienne strips
- 1 pepper, of any color, sown and finely chopped
- 1 cup of peas or peas, cut and cut in half
- 2 tablespoons of chopped chives
- 1 cup of chopped cabbage, spinach or lettuce
- 1 avocado, finely chopped
- 2 tablespoons of chopped cashews

DRESSED

- 1 tablespoon of grated fresh ginger
- 2 tablespoons of cashew butter or almond butter or sunflower seeds
- 2 tablespoons of rice vinegar or apple cider vinegar
- 2 tablespoons of tamari or soy sauce
- 1 teaspoon of toasted sesame oil

143

2-3 tablespoons of water (optional)

1   Boil a medium pot of water and add the pasta Keep it low in the boil, lowering the heat and adding cold water if necessary to keep it cooking .It will take 6 to 7 minutes to cook and sometimes they mix to make sure they don't stick or stick to the bottom of the pot .After cooking, strain into a colander and rinse with hot or cold water, depending on whether you want a hot or cold bowl.

2   You can have raw vegetables, in which case you just have to cut them If you want to cook them, heat a pan over medium heat and fry the carrot with a small amount of water, broth, olive oil or sesame oil .When the carrot softens a little, add the pepper Then add the peas and shallots to the fire for a minute before turning off the heat.

3   Prepare a sauce by squeezing the grated ginger to obtain its juice, then mix all the ingredients or crush them in a small blender, if necessary add 2-3 tablespoons of water to obtain a creamy consistency Put it aside.

4   Arrange the bowl, starting with a layer of chopped cabbage or spinach (for spicy spaghetti) or lettuce (for cold spaghetti), then sprinkle with other tamari and then vegetables.

5   On top, salsa, chopped avocado and a pinch of chopped cashews.

Prepare in advance: cooked and rinsed soba noodles are well stored in the refrigerator, so **prepare** a complete package and keep it handy to quickly transport bowls or lunches for a week

Taco salad with black beans

Make 3 portions

Preparation time: 15 minutes / Cooking time: 5 minutes

RAPID   REINFORCEMENT   RAPID
IMMUNE REINFORCEMENT

Get the full flavor of tacos in a fresh and simple bean salad. I gave you enough mix of black bean taco for three servings. Taste the portion as a salad bowl, then put another in a slightly heated whole bowl Or eat a small bowl of black beans as a snack with tortilla chips. Only part of the black bean mixture is used in tortilla and bowl recipes.

BLACK BEAN SALAD
+   **1 can (14 ounces) of black beans, drained and rinsed, or 1 ½ cup of cooking**
+   **1 cup of corn, fresh and steamed, or frozen and thawed**
+   **¼ cup of fresh coriander or chopped parsley**
+ **1 zest and lime juice**
+   **1-2 teaspoons of chili powder**
+   **A pinch of sea salt**
+   **1½ cup of cherry tomatoes, cut in half**
+ **1 chopped hot pepper**
+ **2 chopped chives**
+   **FOR 1 PORTION OF TORTILLA French fries**
+   **1 large tortilla or whole dish**
+   **1 teaspoon of olive oil**
+   **A pinch of sea salt**
+   **A pinch of freshly ground black pepper**
+   **A pinch of dried oregano**
      A pinch of chilli powder

FOR 1 BOWL
+   **1 cup of fresh vegetables (lettuce, spinach or whatever you want)**

- ¾ cup of cooked quinoa or brown rice, millet or other whole grains
-
- ¼ cup chopped avocado or guacamole
  ¼ cup fresh mango sauce

TO MAKE A BLACK WHEAT SALAD

Mix all the ingredients in a large bowl.

TO MAKE TORTILLA POTATOES

Spread the tortilla with olive oil, then sprinkle with salt, pepper, oregano, chilli powder and other spices .Cut into eight like pizza Transfer the pieces of tortilla to a small baking tray lined with parchment and place them in an oven or toaster on toast or cook for 3-5 minutes, until golden brown .Pay attention to them, because they can quickly change from ready to burned.

CREATE CUENCO

Place the vegetables in a bowl, cover with cooked quinoa, ⅓ black bean salad, avocado and salsa.

Progress: the black bean mixture is especially known if you prepare it in advance, so the flavors have time to mix and merge Store leftovers in the refrigerator in an airtight container .

conclusion

Try this plan for a while and observe the benefits. I always wish you the best, thank you for your trust.

CPSIA information can be obtained
at www.ICGtesting.com
Printed in the USA
BVHW070859150321
602550BV00010B/1096

9 781678 081119